AF379891

Navigating the Code

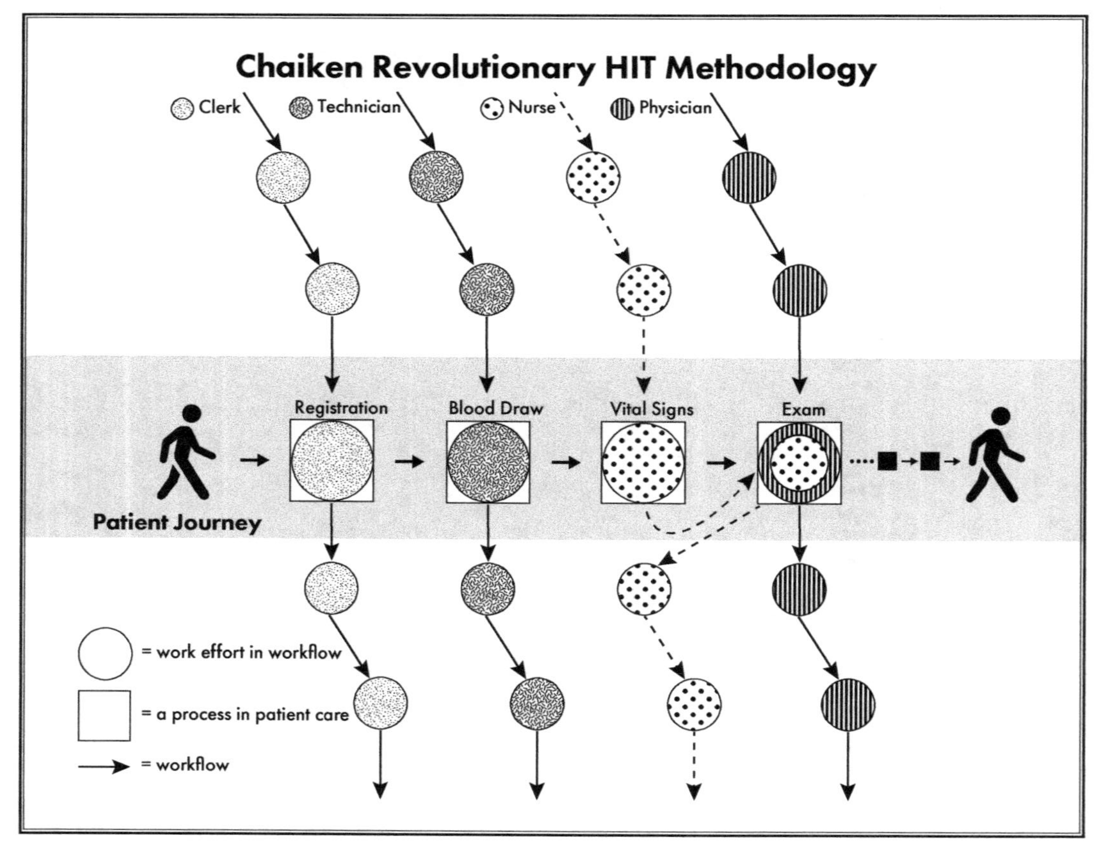

Chaiken Revolutionary HIT Methodology
Clerk
Technician
Nurse
Physician
Registration
Blood Draw
Vital Signs
Exam
Patient Journey
= work effort in workflow
= a process in patient care
= workflow

Navigating the Code

How Revolutionary Technology Transforms the Patient-Physician Journey

Barry P. Chaiken

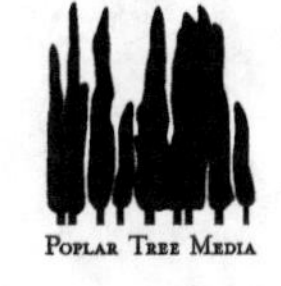

Poplar Tree Media

Boston

Barry P. Chaiken
Poplar Tree Media
14 Durham Street
Boston MA 02115-5301
www.poplartreemedia.com
bchaiken@docsnetwork.com

Cover Design by Christopher Cote

Book Design by Barry P Chaiken

All interview photos are courtesy of those inerviewed.

Hardcover ISBN: 978-1-7367021-2-3 (Black and White edition)
Library of Congress Catalog Control Number: 2021938149

To Ernie Seligmann, teacher, role model, and
advisor to the South Shore High School
student newspaper *Shorelines*, who positively
changed the trajectory of so many lives,
including my own
and
To public education, for giving me the skills to
thrive in my life and career.

Contents

John Halamka, MD, MS, President
The Mayo Clinic Platform

In my 40 years in the healthcare IT industry, I've written a great deal about disruption. I've described the perfect storm when the government, academia and industry align to adopt a new technology.

I've examined the technologies, policies, and psychology of innovation dissemination. If you strip away the bits and bytes, the hype cycle, and the regulatory compliance drivers, the best revolutions in healthcare IT happen with successful change management.

In this book, Dr. Barry Chaiken presents all the tools that clinicians, administrators, and businesspeople need to transform their healthcare organizations with the strategic use of technology.

He does not focus on any one emerging technology—this is not a treatise about cloud, mobile, internet of things, AI, or blockchain. He focuses on the principles that enable organizational transformation regardless of the tech stack.

When I was a graduate student at MIT in the early 1990s,

Professor Hal Abelson taught me that although technology evolves rapidly, engineering concepts stay constant - such as creating systems with modular components that are easily swapped/replaced. It's critical that a book about revolutionary healthcare IT focus on change and the management of change, rather than adoption of any one new product.

Dr. Chaiken's approach is a mixture of core management ideas taken from the past 100 years of leadership literature, with the healthcare domain's specific goals of quality, safety, and efficiency. The book presents a "bedside consultation" in each chapter to ensure the reader has the historical and situational background of the key concepts that are foundational to leading change in healthcare. Chapters are interspersed with interviews/case studies that provide real-world insights from those who have experience in digitizing healthcare.

You can be assured that this is not a text about programming, economic modeling, or navigating regulations. It's a book that synthesizes decades of experience in healthcare leadership into five thematically related sections. The book progresses from the current state of healthcare worldwide to the 21st-century healthcare we need and want.

Along the journey, the reader is treated to the best thinking from Peter Drucker, Avedis Donabedian, and many others.

One of the most remarkable aspects of the book is its multi-disciplinary content. By bringing together such diverse topics as the foundational medical record thinking of Larry Weed, stories about Elon Musk, and even quotes from "Star Trek," the book is extremely readable.

When I write about change, I reflect on personal experiences in my life that have gone well and others that have required me to pick myself up and try a new approach. I tell my students and colleagues that I've made enough mistakes as an IT leader that I know what not to do. I have a sense of guardrails and risk mitigations. I've participated in numerous Harvard Business School cases that highlight my missteps so that others will not repeat them. In this book, Dr. Chaiken synthesizes his own experiences and the wisdom of countless past/current leaders so the reader is handed a roadmap to successful navigation of the change ahead.

Every week at Mayo Clinic I write a "weekly update," summarizing my meetings and progress into a thematic context. I recently summarized my experience leading disruption in healthcare information technology as "navigating without a map." You know where you want to go, but don't know how to get there. In such situations, you must rely on guiding principles and experience. Think of *Navigating the Code: How Revolutionary Technology Transforms the Patient-Physician Journey* as providing both. Armed with the experience of those who have come before (the literal translation of the word "sensei") and principles that put the patient first, the reader has the necessary tools to lead the journey ahead.

The Hippocratic Code

"No sooner are these questions (of patient diagnosis) agitated then the inquirer (a student of medicine) finds fresh difficulties. He has to ask himself, 'What is the standard of success by which I am to judge of the relative value of treatment?' Two replies to this query suggest themselves, viz., the *mortality* from certain diseases and the *duration* of those complaints which are not fatal to life. Ere, however, he can prosecute these ideas, the student finds himself in the presence of another difficulty—he does not know the natural mortality or duration of disease if left alone; and still further, he is positively without any data, whether, in any particular case under treatment, the symptoms of disease and its duration are due to Nature alone, or to the interference of the doctor with her [patient]."

—From the Preface to *The Foundation for a New Theory and Practice of Medicine*, by Thomas Inman, MD
Published by John Churchill, London, in 1861

Hippocrates will likely stand forever at the head of the medical profession, although very little of his original thought is genuinely extant. Even his greatest aphorism, *do no wrong*, is thought to be from the lips of Thomas Inman, a nineteenth-century English surgeon. Although long in the tooth, the remark is exemplary, even if having been reappropriated by Google in its early days.

It would be ill-advised to ignore the basic tenets of the practice of medicine attributed to Hippocrates, and later formulated as the Hippocratic Oath and subsequent Hippocratic Corpus of teachings. It is foundational, yet medicine has changed in every single aspect since Hippocrates lived and administered it in the Golden Age of Greece. The country doctor of just a hundred or so years ago, working from his home office, could not have envisioned the range and depth of changes in today's human healthcare.

Even if we look back only as far as the early 2000s at *House*, the television doctor and his staff thinking and talking their way through a patient's illness, stumbling from one diagnosis to another without benefit of computers, we would be hard-pressed to appreciate just how profoundly computer technology has impacted the medical profession. But changes have also occurred throughout medical practice, even encompassing its branding: now termed healthcare, to reflect the fact that medicine is today not only concerned with healing the ill and diseased but also with sustaining the well-being of the healthy.

What the healthcare industry may have overlooked is the growing enormity of its own significance. The twentieth century saw the greatest increase in world population in human history, rising to over six billion from 1.6 billion. Meanwhile, the United States failed to address the growing needs of the aging baby-boomer generation, which put vastly more people into the healthcare system than had previous generations. As a result of these and other factors, today's healthcare is having trouble keeping up. Emergency departments

(ED) are often the waiting room for non-emergency healthcare because there is no other designated place for them. Hospitals have either outgrown or reallocated their physical facilities, resulting in fewer beds. Burned-out, overworked doctors and nurses are fleeing the profession. By their claims-handling, payers are contributing to the dehumanization of the most human-centered of professions. The list goes on and on, but the bottom line is, healthcare is growing ever more out of step with social needs or a sustainable business model for itself. It is swamped with patients it cannot handle, rising costs, declining profits, ever greater pressure to comply with business and governmental policies and requirements. Here are just a few of the major issues confronting the healthcare business today:

- The spend today is greater than it was for similar outcomes previously.

- There are more complex patient problems, diagnoses, and treatments.

- Best practices based upon evidence-based care are not universally followed, although there is no reason why they should not be.

- Healthcare variance on outcomes is too great.

- Outcomes should be uniformly appraised, both by treatment and by cost; in other words, the care received in Boston should not be at great variance from that received in Lake Placid or even rural Wyoming.

Much of this the clinician may unfortunately already know and understand. Yet the reality of these statistics was brutally brought home by the recent COVID-19 virus pandemic, which shook every foundation of modern life to its roots: commerce, government, and certainly healthcare. May we never again be so unprepared for such an eventuality.

Former surgeon general Jerome Adams characterized the COVID-19 virus as "our Pearl Harbor, our 9/11, moment," a catastrophic failure of the healthcare system and the government's preparation. We hope the worst of the pandemic phase may be behind us, but we have to accept that we continue to live in difficult, even dangerous times. The pandemic created ripple effects throughout our society, just as so many predicted.

We know this: a degree and proportion of change has hit the world's population and infiltrated the planet's economy like a tsunami. It has fragmented aspects of our lives that were once whole, and it has amalgamated aspects that were once disparate, neither to the benefit of healthcare nor to humankind. All this change has been problematic as we try to readjust to a pandemic-riddled world. Readjust we will, but no one really knows how, or for how long, it will take.

Clearly, we had become over reliant on so many institutions—most importantly healthcare—and that overreliance weakened us individually and collectively. Our urgent penchant for automated systems and processes has, across the board, resulted in our ceding personal involvement and/or intelligent oversight and control over many aspects of our lives. And it has led to a staggering resistance to change; there is a perceived fragility, a resignation, or a "if it is not broke do not fix it" way of thinking about how we work and live our lives. As a result, we are left with our species' greatest gift, adaptability, diminished. Yet we must learn to live and work with the latest buzzword technologies we have created: computer vision, digital dashboards, hyper automation, machine language, "mobile first," quantum computing, and on and on. The bottom line for healthcare professionals: we must make all of it work more productively and appropriately for the good of our patients.

Change and adaptation are often at the forefront of how we think about and view life. Yet, odd as it might sound, they are only infrequently the way we practice life and work. They have certainly become highly held principles for today's patient care, and possess another type of special role with respect to healthcare information technology (HIT) systems. In more instances than can be enumerated, HIT has created, driven, and implemented significant, essential change in healthcare, while facilitating our adaptation to new and more efficient ways of working. The what, why, and how of managing HIT is paramount to effecting change and adaptation within healthcare. Yet it is my opinion that we do not manage or take advantage of HIT as much as we could, which is to say we do not practice change and adaptation well.

As Dylan George, a former Obama administration official at the White House Office of Science and Technology Policy, said on *60 Minutes*, "Data and technology transformed the way we do business and many aspects of our lives, but it has not transformed the way things are done in public health." Yet, in the post-pandemic era, it has become paramount that we do so. Greater change and inevitable adaption lie before us. They have always been, but in these uncertain times they must be factored into a healthcare organization's critical success practices. Simply put, that means HIT becomes the driving force for effecting change management and organizational adaptation.

Author and LSU business professor Leon C. Megginson once wrote, "It is not the strongest of the species that survives, nor the most intelligent. It is the one that is most adaptable to change." This is what this book intends to address. In order to do so, I wish to refamiliarize the reader with the fundamentals of healthcare, the basic tenets by which all healthcare is ostensibly practiced by all of its practitioners. With all due respect to the title of Dan Brown's popular novel, I characterize them as the Hippocratic Code.

The Hippocratic Code: Rediscovering Healthcare Basics

If Hippocrates lived today, I believe he would propound a basic set of ethical and behavioral guidelines—a code, if you will—by which healthcare ought to be practiced. Although new in this particular form of expression, these basics were central to classical Greek philosophical thought, as well as to other early Ayurveda or Islamic practices of medicine. The code is based on four simple tenets: quality and safety, access, outcomes, and the resulting cost of healthcare.

Every patient and every healthcare professional has these basic deliverables in mind for every patient transaction. It may be fair to say they have been slighted or overlooked on occasion, but they have remained immutable. Yet what we see all around us today is change and change management, in large part due to the ever-increasing integration of information technology with healthcare. The process of delivering these basics has often unintentionally fallen to the wayside because of automation—and in some cases because of a lack of automation—but they have never been forgotten. Let us take a closer look at quality and safety, access, outcomes, and the resulting costs associated with twenty-first-century healthcare.

First, the quality of healthcare services while ensuring patient safety in the process;

Second, access to healthcare, and determining its outcomes;

Third, outcomes that are satisfactory to both clinician and patient; and

Fourth, an *investment-responsible* process that benefits the patient, healthcare provider, and society, and that can be managed to assure successful outcomes.

Henceforth throughout this book, I will replace the term *cost* with *investment-responsible.* Simply put, we need to shift our considering patient care and outcomes an *expense* to an *investment,* one benefiting both the patient and the provider. We need to recognize that a successful outcome truly accrues value to both.

When all four are performed at the highest levels of expertise, they collectively deliver what I term superior outcomes. When this is the end result of the delivery system, it is inherently efficient, cost-effective, and will satisfy the patient's needs.

Quality and safety. Quality care is the result of the patient-clinician transaction: one, the quality of the clinical outcomes, and two, the quality of the experience. The quality of the outcome is determined by the problem and how it was diagnosed, cited, and resolved, using the best possible practices known to the clinician on behalf of the patient. That said, the clinician also benefits by knowing she has used best practices, established procedures, and appropriate functionality for diagnosis and treatment, whether a sore throat or cancer. By expressing concern and care for the patient's experience during the treatment phase, along with a level of professional service that was satisfying and corrective, the clinician has gained more and better experience and satisfying outcomes.

Usually, both patient and clinician are in a stressful situation in any medical intervention, and the pace at which healthcare is administered can make this intimate human-to-human experience impersonal. The clinician's task is to make the service as easy, uncomplicated, and seamless as possible. From a care and even a marketing perspective, we often refer to this as the patient experience. Without doubt, the patient should be made to feel well treated and cared for. Equally important is the other side of the patient experience, and that has to do with the data collected and its usefulness after the transaction. How so?

The clinician cannot manage any of the diagnostic and treatment processes essential to delivering quality care unless they are measured. They must be recorded and tracked to make it possible to understand them—simply put, to see what worked and what did not—and to make changes based on results as well as what patients liked or did not about the care they received.

Patient safety must always accompany quality care as an equally primary concern. Safety is tied to quality in many ways, clearly because it assures patients do not have bad outcomes. Any medical process provides treatment and safety structure to healthcare delivery, but bad outcomes result from not following established processes or choosing to use untested or ad hoc processes. And if the impact of a process is not measured, it cannot be satisfactorily changed or modified when it delivers an unintended or unsatisfactory outcome. This was the great failure of the out-of-date "cookbook medicine" methodology, based on rigid protocols rather than informed processes. Often the clinician, due to a lack of training or other human factors, fails to achieve a minimum level of success. The unproven process gets in the way of delivering good care. The bad process, of course, delivers substandard (or worse) outcomes and assures inferior and unsatisfactory care. It is quite difficult to produce a satisfactory and consistent level of quality outcomes when established, tested, and measured processes are not in place.

For example, an internist accedes to a prescription change at the patient's insistence, even though the drug in use has not been administered for the prescribed length of time to be effective. Or say the nurse-practitioner forgets to give the patient a printed copy of the office visit or post-surgery procedures. Failing to follow established procedures happens, but in order to assure it only does so rarely, and in order to achieve the highest levels of healthcare delivery, demands HIT's involvement. In these cases it is a simple enough checkbox on the tablet's screen that automatically prints instructions and sends a copy electronically, as well as updating the patient's app or portal. That is too much like a protocol punch list. What the human healthcare clinician might forget, the HIT does not.

Access. From a healthcare IT perspective, access is about capacity management (CM). CM design assures your organization can handle varying care demands of patients. For example, you do not want patients to have to wait for cancer therapy or inflamed gallbladder removal. Some procedures require staged visits both prior to and following an intervention, yet if the patient is acutely ill, you want to get them into the workflow as quickly as possible. Patients cannot get healthcare if they cannot access healthcare.

CM resources are the centerpiece. Without adequate staff, equipment, facilities, and an IT infrastructure to manage these resources, you cannot achieve successful healthcare access. The patient experience initiates all workflow and its processes. Post-procedure is when we can measure the overall outcomes. You must possess an understanding of what outcomes are expected and, indeed, unanticipated, then be prepared to initiate alternative processes as the situation requires. It is not just about the system functionality, nor whether the patient was healed or cured. For example, how long was the hospital stay? Was it consistent with predicated benchmarks? If it was longer, why, and how ought that be addressed? Are you satisfied with the outcome?

CM is essential for assessing outcomes. Foremost, was the patient's experience data collected and analyzed? Failing to ask for feedback means that you cannot effectively learn the appropriate lessons from the process. The clinician or the facility must have a constant feedback flow from patients.

Another strategic outcome is assuring that all the people, equipment, and supplies are on hand to provide the patient treatment. Again, HIT can make the difference between success and failure by tracking these process elements, whether they are things that are obvious, such as sutures or cotton balls, or things that are not, such as a patient stuck in a prep room for three hours because a critical staff member had called in sick.

It goes without saying that all of the above are essential for capacity planning, which is the first step in capacity management. And capacity planning is essential to your organizational success. That simply means the outcomes, both good and bad, must be analyzed and deliberated, then appropriate adjustments made in processes and workflows. The nurse who had to sit with the patient awaiting care for three hours cost the organization three hours of her salary and expertise, which ought to have been spent doing her real job.

If your HIT is not capturing this detailed level of data—or if you are, but you are not processing it as CM data that can be linked to the organization's prescribed outcomes—then it is useless data. You are flying blind and you will have great difficulty improving your organizational proficiency. You will not know if your services are achieving satisfactory outcomes for your patients. You will not know which doctors are exemplary or which are in need of more training, support, or motivation. This is a CM adjustment strategy: we face an ongoing shortage of doctors and nurses, so this is a praise-in-public, remonstrate-in-private moment for the chief of staff. The way to improve healthcare is to maximize capacity planning and integrate it with efficient scheduling of people and physical resources, all of which can be best accomplished with the participation of HIT.

Outcomes. Ask any clinician and they will say that an outcome is, preferably, the successful treatment of a patient's illness or completion of the applied medical intervention. It is far too common for the physician, and often the patient as well, to be somewhat uncertain about the outcome of a procedure. This is because the outcome is commonly the product of the clinician's experience and intuition. While these perceptions are often spot-on and should never be discounted or discarded, with today's advanced technology it is much to our advantage to use the vast amount of computer-based data to aid us in our quest for better and more predictable outcomes.

An outcome is not just clinical; it is administrative as well. The diagnosis, the administrative requisition for treatment, and the outcome must be identical. If there is variance, it must be acknowledged clinically, represented in procedure orders, and dealt with as an antecedent to the outcome. Every step must be identified, processed, and accounted for. The use of computerized data collection and representation is of significant utility in doing so.

Investment responsible cost. We live in a rather ethereal world where many enterprises operate at a loss year after year, ever waiting for the hoped-for turnaround. Healthcare cannot operate in this manner. Similarly, hospitals often do not know the true costs of their healthcare services, and as a result have no sense of what they should charge for them, which, of course, means they do not have a sound grasp on their P&L.

Although hospitals have been reported as overcharging for their services at an average rate of *three and a half to fifteen* times cost—even though private payers intentionally overpay reimbursements to help keep them solvent and subsidize government budgets—and although less than 4 percent of U.S. hospital costs remain uncompensated for, hospitals across the board make only about 8 percent in profit, two points lower than the national average of 10 percent. To coin a phrase, they are living from paycheck to paycheck. The COVID-19 pandemic has placed even greater strains on budgets. The CDC estimates the morbidity for victims of COVID-19 to commonly last three to six weeks, depending on age and general health, which takes staff out of the workforce and puts them in the hospital for indefinite periods of time.

The problem is not so much that hospital profits are low; rather, the problem is that they need to overhaul their cost accounting practices. Business data analysis and feedback loops must extend into financial management, in much the same manner that capacity planning is managed. Practitioners and administrators alike must become the guardians and champions of the P&L, asking the tough questions and getting forthright answers that will help create more businesslike outcomes. Likert scale questionnaires are popular and powerful because they are simple to use and produce useful data. The physicians, nurses, clinical support staff, and certainly patients—anyone who is in the workflow and processes—should be asked for their experience, opinions, and suggestions for improvement.

Cost, or investment, is most effectively driven by process and evidence-based care—not the other way around. These can be measured, and they must be if you are to really understand how healthcare works. All the tools required to gather, measure, and understand the applicable data, and effect the necessary changes, are probably available right now from your institution's HIT. But you might need to ask for what you want.

There is nothing hierarchical about these four mission-critical Hippocratic Code tenets of effective healthcare. Quality of care and safety, access, outcomes, and investment responsibility must be managed as an objective of healthcare service delivery, even when the P&L sheet reads like a Stephen King novel. And they cannot be managed for success without the grassroots involvement of HIT.

Healthcare is a business. Using HIT's advanced software tools helps you make better business decisions, just as in every other enterprise on earth. They can lead you to discover new paths, new research, and better solutions. They can help you deliver the invest-ment-responsible care you want to provide, while guiding you away from doing things that are costly, harmful, counterproductive, or a waste of time to either patient or provider.

This is the most important point I wish to make in this book. I am certain your organization has a HIT department. How well do you understand its services and its mission? In how many ways could it be doing a better job for you, your staff, your department, your institution? Do you feel as though HIT is your partner in solving problems, supporting processes, and improving workflow?

If you are nodding and chanting, "I need help with all of the above and more," then your HIT is in need of a revolution. The truth is, most HIT organizations are. Revolutionary healthcare informa-tion technology (RHIT), well implemented, can bring the essential change management to help healthcare out of its morass. Most HIT organizations keep the back office running smoothly. Revolutionary HIT offers clinicians, researchers, and administrators immensely powerful tools to drive clinical and administrative processes so your organization can deliver high-quality, safe, accessible, and invest-ment-responsible medical care for a rapidly changing world.

Back in the late 1970s and early 1980s, most large enterprises began to realize that IT was not the organization's mechanics but rather its engineers. This led to a lot of dramatic change in the relationship between the computer guys and the business guys. The appellation "MIS" (management information system) for the com-puter department emerged. It portended the relationship change: we must work together to solve business problems with technology.

As this book and those quoted here make clear, our global healthcare systems, one and all, are in need of change on a revolutionary scale. Healthcare, without attributing blame, has not kept pace with other large enterprises, whether for-profit or not. I am not talking about an overthrow, but rather something more on the order of a phoenix bird rising from the ashes. What is needed is the change management leadership and the strategies to do so. Perhaps, like the poet William Blake's "fearful symmetry," a new defining of the relationship between healthcare delivery services and HIT is in order. For this, we need a full deployment of the HIT troops. Revolutionary HIT can be a significant part of the solution, which we will describe in detail throughout the following pages.

The more you practice healthcare that encompasses these four Hippocratic Code tenets—quality, access, outcomes, and investment—the more you refine and improve your reiterative processes. The result is improved quality, more efficient access, and better financial management. You will find yourself doing more with less and producing better outcomes.

Read on.

The Road to RHIT

"I have curiosity. I'm always looking for a paradox, or information that adds to or contradicts my beliefs. . . . I want to be governed by people who are much smarter than I am."

—John Cleese

When I began my medical career as a medical detective at the Centers for Disease Control more than twenty-five years ago, my technology tools were a stethoscope and a blood pressure cuff. Our information came primarily from paper reports and attending conferences. Computers were for the back-office accounting and management staff, not for doctors.

Look at the progress we have made.

Or have we?

Of course we have. As the famed science-fiction author Arthur C. Clarke, who penned the novel *2001: A Space Odyssey*, said so well, "Any sufficiently advanced technology is indistinguishable from magic." It would be interesting to know just how many lives we have saved in modern healthcare because we were able to employ advanced technology.

My interest in the magic of technology has paralleled my medical pursuits. They were the two hands washing each other. Yet over the years I saw healthcare failing to sufficiently take advantage of technology. We seemed to get to a place where the prevailing attitude was "good enough" use of high tech. That was no surprise; it was a fact established in the late 1980s that humans would recall no more than seven functions of a technology tool, for example how to save, copy, footnote, or change from sum to count. Those few who mastered more were called "power users."

This book is about how practicing clinicians all ought to become power users. We must raise our sights to how much more we can achieve through expanding our technological knowledge and skills in the practice of healthcare. We are not doing badly; witness our continuing recovery from the 2020 pandemic. But there is so much more we could be doing if we were only to deploy all the technological tools at our disposal.

Years ago, I came up with a name for this quantum movement forward in our profession: *revolutionary healthcare*. I realized the best—perhaps the only—way to take the necessary next steps in delivering health alongside treating symptoms was with more technology. I began referring to this solution as healthcare information technology (HIT), to which I added the term *revolutionary*, hence the use of the term *revolutionary technology* in the subtitle of this book.

To that phrase I honed and refined the following description:

Revolutionary Healthcare Information Technology (RHIT) offers clinicians, researchers, and administrators immensely powerful tools to drive clinical and administrative processes to deliver high-quality, safe, accessible, and investment-responsible medical outcomes.

Note that I include administrators in my definition. We need the admin people to keep our business and our partnerships with payers and governmental agencies intact and thriving. There may be misunderstandings and some friction at times, but the clinical-administrative relationship must be cared for as rigorously as the clinician-patient relationship.

The RHIT platform. From this platform, if I may call it that, over time I defined the six main concerns I believe all of us in healthcare—both clinicians and administrators—must focus on for constant improvement.

1. More time with the patient. This is job number one. I call it the human touch and it should never be left to an indifferent payer to determine the amount of time or care spent with patients.

2. Computers have no "bedside manner." They are essential, but their purpose is to support healthcare. Tasks computers are good at should be handled by computers; patient care is what doctors and nurses are best at, and should be respected first and foremost.

3. Workflows are how each of us gets our jobs done. Processes guide all of our workflows toward our institutional objective. When clinical and administrative workflows are in sync, we have effective, efficient, business process management.

4. Good business process management is always the result of implementing healthcare information technology.

5. Better integration of HIT makes better outcomes more consistently possible.

6. *Revolutionary healthcare information technology* (RHIT) uses analytics to improve processes, facilitates evidence-based medicine at the point of care, and affirms the workflows to guide clinicians to the best outcomes.

Over time I developed a model and a visualization of this, which I call the Chaiken RHIT Methodology. It is presented in Chapter 5 and is integrated into discussions throughout the book. The Chaiken RHIT Methodology uses analytics to assess pertinent data and guide the patient to a successful outcome. Metrics assigned to a particular process allow us to evaluate, learn from, and then iterate meaningful change within that process for the highest quality of care and a repurposed focus on successful outcomes. I believe this emphasis creates more efficient processes and workflows and leads to a sound investment, which we all believe is necessary for healthcare to improve.

Such a system enhances the essence of healthcare. It is the product of an optimistic, empowering, positive, people-centered business model that puts the relationship between the clinicians and the patients front and center, assuring trust, with the solid backing and support from essential administrative services.

Navigating the Code intends to demonstrate that these goals and objectives are achievable without tossing out the existing system, but rather by developing some new ways of thinking about workflows and processes.

How *Navigating the Code* Is Structured

Navigating the Code consists of five Parts:

Part I: Thinking about Healthcare (Chapters 1 through 4) provides an overview of today's healthcare environment.

Part II: Transforming Today's Healthcare with Revolutionary HIT (Chapters 5 through 8) disseminates the business aspects of healthcare with an emphasis on its information technology and the need to revolutionize it in the quest for an overall transformation of our business operations.

Part III: Applied Change Management (Chapters 9 through 12) begins with a basic introduction to personal and institutional change, followed by in-depth explorations of change management for IT, workflow, clinicians, and, last but not least, patients.

Part IV: Revolutionary HIT (Chapters 13 through 17) returns to the key theme of the book, revolutionary healthcare information technology. The degree of change needed to restructure healthcare cannot be accomplished without a revolution throughout the organization; these five chapters explain how and why in detail.

Part V: True Twenty-First-Century Healthcare (Chapters 18 and 19) sums up by stating we have not achieved any significant changes to our business in the twenty-first century, and goes on to explain how we can begin making the decisions and taking the necessary steps to achieve transformative healthcare.

Chapters have been written at a length appropriate for reading in a single sitting. I encourage you to highlight, underline, and otherwise annotate as you read to frame questions and enhance your understanding.

Throughout the book, you will find two features:

- Bedside Consult, exemplary anecdotes apropos of the chapter theme, and

- The RHIT Interview, interviews I have personally conducted with healthcare professionals from all around the world who share many differing perspectives on healthcare.

Both are intended to give you a perspective that I alone could not. I hope they enhance your interest in learning what is possible for the future of healthcare.

PART I

Thinking about Healthcare

There is a classic line from Bob Dylan's "Subterranean Homesick Blues" that goes, "I'm on the pavement, thinking about the government."

In my case, I find myself sitting in front of my computer, thinking about the worldwide healthcare industry. A distinctly human behavior is to procrastinate about most everything, in our case the state of healthcare. Of course the COVID-19 pandemic shook healthcare to its foundations, and there have been many changes instituted since it was unleashed upon us. But they are Band-Aids, addressing specific issues or problems. They do not address systemic change that will improve our entire industry, from soup to nuts. That is what I propose in this book. The first four chapters assess where we are:

- Chapter 1 looks at healthcare and its social impact on life on planet Earth.

- Chapter 2 introduces healthcare information technology and its role.

- Chapter 3 takes a close look at our greatest challenge, managing change.

- Chapter 4 is a surgeon's-eye view of how healthcare works today and why it needs systemic change.

This, then, is what I have been observing and thinking about for many years. I hope you share my concerns and are reading this book to learn how you can help change healthcare.

Chapter 1

The Current State of Worldwide Healthcare

> "Life is difficult. This is a great truth, one of the greatest truths. It is a great truth because once we truly see this truth, we transcend it."
>
> —M. Scott Peck, MD, PhD, *The Road Less Traveled*

What is the current state of worldwide healthcare? Simply put, it is fraught with more problems than it can, under present circumstances and using present means, hope to solve. If you work in healthcare, you already understand this. You feel this discomfort and frustration on a daily basis. These are endemic problems, difficult to solve, that will not be fixed with the proverbial silver bullet. But they can be fixed.

Among our most challenging problems:

- *The ongoing COVID-19 pandemic.* It has been compared to the stock market crash of 1929 in terms of its economic impact. Even though this book is being published long after its initial event horizon, the aftereffects are still with us now and will be for many years. Its emotional scars will create a ripple effect the scope of a tidal wave, and in that respect our current healthcare crisis is on a par with the last World War. If there had been any doubt, the pandemic of 2020 proved that healthcare is the most mission-critical industry in the world. Without a sufficient healthcare workforce, all enterprises and economies around the world will suffer: Belarus experienced its greatest economic decline in over twenty-five years; Portugal saw a decline in GNP of at least 6.9 percent; in the U.S., the pandemic was out of control in every one of the forty-eight contiguous states for many months. Only time and massive amounts of data collection will reveal in what ways, and just how seriously, the impact will be for the world at large.

- *A rapidly aging population.* The baby-boomer generation presents one of the most formidable challenges to the healthcare industry. According to a World Health Organization (WHO) 2019 report, the number of people aged sixty years or older was a billion, and is estimated to double by the year 2050—an "unprecedented pace." In the U.S. alone, population growth is anticipated to grow to 420 million by 2060, half of which will be minorities by 2043. Growth in Middle Eastern countries will increase at rates as high as 3 percent. Worldwide, the need for healthcare services will fill doctors' offices like a Taylor Swift concert hall.

- *A looming shortage of both doctors and nurses.* In 2020, largely in part due to the effects of the COVID-19 pandemic, hundreds of hospitals closed their doors, or were acquired, for financial reasons. By 2030, the shortage of doctors will top 120,000. We cannot afford to have fewer places where care is dispensed. Healthcare in the United States is big business: It is the fourth largest industry in the U.S. It accounts for three trillion dollars, or 18 percent, of the national U.S. Gross Domestic Product (GDP). Yet it is not so large that its back cannot break.

Even now, we can only hope to recover and restore some vestige of our healthcare industry to sustainable patient satisfaction, productivity, and profit. This book is intended to point the direction to take toward those goals by making the case for increased and vastly improved collaboration between healthcare administration, clinical services, and information technology. In these pages I present a solution: how these collaborationists can deploy my revolutionary healthcare information technology (RHIT) tools and processes, and the strategies they will need to make healthcare better. Each of us must do our part. It cannot happen unless clinicians and those supporting clinical services take up the mantle of change and adaptation.

- *The healthcare balance sheet does not reconcile.* Inherent in every medical intervention is a value-based transaction. That includes the investment made by the patient and the provider, represented by the treatment they receive and its outcome. The *perceived* value of the intervention as well as the investment must correlate with the value paid. This is the deepest value imbalance in healthcare, and it reaches from patient-physician all the way to the costs and profits of the entire industry. No consumer would buy an auto with only three wheels and say, "good enough," and the same value proposition ought to be inherent in healthcare—except it is not.

The technology conundrum. Healthcare ranks with education as a high-knowledge and technology-intensive (H-KTI) industry, the two assets contributing about 25 percent of the U.S. GDP, the country where it is the greatest. The range of H-KTI devices for healthcare diagnostics and treatments is immense, and growing all the time. Similarly, software advances in data analysis, artificial intelligence, informatics, and telecommunication are becoming more pervasive and complex. Yet the HIT organization is often ignored, underutilized, or poorly guided, when it could be designing a systems infrastructure with more and better technology utilization across the entire healthcare spectrum, from the patient appointment to the use of electronic health records (EHRs) to data analysis and diagnostics and, not least, a profitable administrative backbone.

As a physician myself, I have watched as most of these problems emerged, a multitude of Medusa-like snakes befouling the best, most earnest efforts in healthcare. I have often thought healthcare's problems were like the streets of Boston, where I live. Streets, once cow paths both long and short, came to wend this way or that as the city grew over the past four hundred years into convoluted roundabouts; intersections without traffic lights; one-way streets that only increased congestion; roadways unable to accommodate wider cars, larger trucks, and fragile bicycles. Rush hour in Boston and its surrounding cities is now a never-ending constant.

Although certainly not as charming or romantic as letting yourself get lost in downtown Boston (which, it turns out, is very likely), street-grid traffic made much more sense as witnessed in New York City and Barcelona, both of which intentionally created a grid pattern for their streets as a move away from early unplanned-influenced chaos. And of course that is our point: roadways and most of humankind's other workflows can be designed, analyzed, and improved upon when they are systematized. We thank Henry Ford for designing and creating an assembly line to systematize building cars. For all its other shortcomings, it is better, faster, and cheaper than any other system of industrial mass production.

Like industrial production, most human workflows can be analyzed and redesigned into more efficient systems. So can healthcare. It is just that no one has tried or perhaps thought about how to go about it. Healthcare may be one of our most leading-edge industries, but it is also likely that it is our least well systematized. It is just so complex that it is hard to know where to begin.

Solving that issue is what this book is about. The key to fixing most everything that ails healthcare (if that is not an oxymoron, I do not know what is) can be done by applying a systematized overlay (a grid map, if you will) that encompasses all its activities and aspects and organizes them into a workflow-directed process. "Where will that come from?" you might ask. To which I reply, "Information technology." Your very own healthcare information technology (HIT) people.

Imagining, designing, building, and deploying systems is what IT does, and does well. HIT simply has not been asked to undertake this immense yet essential task. It is far too late to redesign Boston streets, but it certainly is not too late to systematize healthcare. The chapters that follow describe in some detail some of the various issues and problems of healthcare and explore ways in which healthcare administrators, clinicians, clinical support staff, pharmacists, and service and solutions providers can help rescue healthcare from its undifferentiated Medusa-like condition.

Bedside Consult: Great Events in Healthcare History

Solving big problems is nothing new for scientists, researchers, or medical practitioners. They have always known that their mission is to solve knotty problems. Faced with what today seems an insurmountable problem, just remember someone else has faced their own and solved it. Here are a few highlights from the history of medical research, the practice of medicine, and what became known as healthcare. Each of these problem-solvers was troubled by concerns about health and illness, and was emboldened to set upon them to find solutions. As with COVID-19 clinicians, many risked their lives in their studies and pursuits.

Throughout the ages, problem-solvers have asked themselves and others, "What if . . . ?" And although we live in an incredibly new and different era, transformed by technological innovation (and a pandemic), we still ask the simple "what if?" question but more often resolve it with the assistance of a software app. But there it is, and even in its simplest form, it remains a diagnostic tool that has been used by scientists and clinicians for several thousand years. Here are a few to buoy your spirits for the task at hand.

Chinese medicine, similarly to the evolution of medicine in India, was founded on spiritual and metaphysical values, namely Taoism, about four to five thousand years ago. It encompasses acupuncture, ginseng and other herbal medicines, and massage, all of which are utterly alien to practitioners of Western medicine. Chinese medicine propounded a quest to answer the question "why?" and to combine the physical symptoms with mental and spiritual causation.

The *Sushruta Samhita*, dating back to around 300 BCE, may be the first book of medicine to elaborate on surgery, and the workflow of diagnosis and prognosis. It established the foundation for Ayurveda and is thought to be the work of an Indian doctor named Suśruta.

Hippocrates, it turns out, was the given name of an entire family of individuals who were concerned with the study of medicine. The father figure was Hippocrates of Kos (a Greek island) who lived from 460–370 BCE. He is remembered in the West as the father of medicine and founder of the first school of medicine; beyond that, little is known about the man. As mentioned in the Introduction, the Hippocratic Oath was a living document, the product of successive generations of thought, but founded on Hippocrates's principles.

Quintus Serenus Sammonicus, a second-century (CE) Roman man of medicine, is fondly remembered for incanting "Abracadabra" over a patient with a fever.

Galen of Pergamon, another second-century (CE) Roman, wrote a work declaring the best physician was also a philosopher. He is remembered for his studies in anatomy and physiology and for following up on Hippocrates's research into the discovery of the four humors: black bile, yellow bile, blood, and phlegm. But Galen is most notable for codifying the Hippocratic Oath.

A Swiss, Theophrastus von Hohenheim, better known as Paracelsus, was an early Renaissance physician who proposed that observation was as important to diagnosis as established prognosis. He is remembered for his studies and discoveries in liniments, pain relief, syphilis, contracting disease from human contact, and, from his wartime medical experience, septic infections: "If you prevent infection, Nature will heal the wound all by herself."

In 1847, Ignaz Semmelweis, a Hungarian surgeon, told his colleagues that he had a new theory: women giving birth were dying because the administering clinician, having come from performing autopsies covered in blood and gore, was infecting and killing them. His simple solution was for doctors to wash their hands. Semmelweis was laughed at, but was proved correct after his early death (ironically, perhaps the result of an infection). Puerperal fever was eventually eradicated and Semmelweis was crowned "the savior of mothers."

Nineteenth-century Marie Curie, whom we remember as Madame Curie, devoted much of her scientific research to radioactivity, a term that she coined and from which she died. Curie discovered the chemical element polonium, also giving it a name. We can thank her for creating mobile radiography units that provided

X-ray services to soldiers during World War I. Born in Poland, her career thrived in Paris; she founded Curie Institutes in both countries and won the Nobel Prize twice.

Louis Pasteur, another nineteenth-century biologist, a native Frenchman and contemporary of Marie Curie, is best remembered for creating the pasteurization process embodied from his last name. A tireless researcher, he created vaccines for anthrax and rabies, and refined the process of vaccination. Germ theory underscored most of his studies, which, following Paracelsus's lead, proved that contamination spreads disease.

Alexander Fleming, a Scottish doctor, discovered penicillin, the first antibiotic, on moldy bread in 1928. It was later learned that ancient Egyptians made a poultice from moldy bread to heal infected wounds. At the time, he did not see its potential for fighting bacteria like diphtheria and streptococcus. He won the Nobel Prize, was knighted, and named one of the twentieth century's most important people by *Time* magazine.

Experiments in implanting artificial organs began as early as the 1950s. The twentieth century further paved the way for further technological innovation in medicine. In the 1960s, Dr. Lawrence Leonard "Larry" Weed, introduced his problem-oriented medical record format and the subjective, objective assessment plan, or SOAP notes, which became the foundational structure for the EHR. The internet and World Wide Web spawned online medical information from the online zine WebMD and major healthcare providers such as Johns Hopkins and Stanford universities and teaching hospitals such as Mass General Brigham and the Mayo Clinic.

Technological innovation in the twenty-first century so far has been nothing short of astounding. It is occurring at a faster pace than most people and enterprises can assimilate, which is the subject of the next chapter. Organs and body parts printed on a 3-D printer? Computer technology has surely brought more innovation to healthcare than any other industry, even though only a fraction of it is used on a daily basis. Healthcare IT is a sleeping giant.

Amid such technological breakthroughs, we can trace the popular interest in medicine from radio's *Dr. Kildare* to television's *Grey's Anatomy* or *House*, and the many recent documentaries. Throughout, the challenges posed to medicine, and how it is practiced, continue growing exponentially. We need only look at the rise and might of the allied pharmaceutical business to see how far we have come from "take two aspirin and call me in the morning."

Healthcare Challenges

Healthcare is undoubtedly one of our most complex industries. It has so many inputs, outputs, and interstitial connections into the lives of its clientele, the roles of its workforce, and its impact upon life as we know it. Yet prepare for the future it must, because each country and the world depend upon it making a good job of it. There are solutions, and they exist now, awaiting recognition and implementation. The two keys to unlock the solutions are change and adaptation, subjects we will return to again and again in this book.

Change. It goes without saying that twenty-first-century healthcare is our country's most challenged—and challenging—industry, beset upon by disparate forces from all sides. Having said it anyway, acknowledging the situation needs to become the *cri de coeur* of healthcare. There must be a call to action, each to his or her chosen specialty. Doctors have a reputation for being resistant to change, for a variety of reasons. As author Dr. M. Scott Peck wrote:

"Human beings are poor examiners, subject to superstition, bias, prejudice, and a profound tendency to see what they want to see rather than what is really there."

We all must change.

Adaptability. Change and adaptability go hand in hand. After the COVID-19 pandemic began, a great deal of press dialogue concerned how our lives would never be the same. That has been borne out as true. There is so much change and adaptability ahead for the healthcare profession that it seems like an insurmountable challenge to what we do, what we stand for, and how we are perceived by the general public. This is precisely why we must change and develop our own acute-care natural selection process for our work and our industry.

We must change as individuals. We must change our healthcare processes. We must work as hard as we can to remove inefficiencies, disorder, randomness, indeed chaos, from our workflow. There are so many changes ahead of us—replacing undisciplined, unscientific medical-care delivery with fully realized, data-driven healthcare, the shift away from episodic medical practice to a value-based delivery system, ultimately an interoperable EHR platform. All of these are industry game changers, and we must develop a heart that embraces change and sinews of adaptability to embrace and implement it when it occurs.

There is no way we can allow ourselves to go the way of the buggy whip or the dinosaur. Charles Darwin, writing in *On the Origin of Species*, put it this way:

"It is not the most intellectual of the species that survives;
it is not the strongest that survives; but the species that
survives is the one that is able to adapt to and to adjust
best to the changing environment in which it finds itself."

The RHIT Interview: Beatriz de Faria-Leao, MD, PhD, at the Universidade Federal de São Paulo, Brazil

1. What was the most significant event or factor that determined your pursuing a career in healthcare information technology?

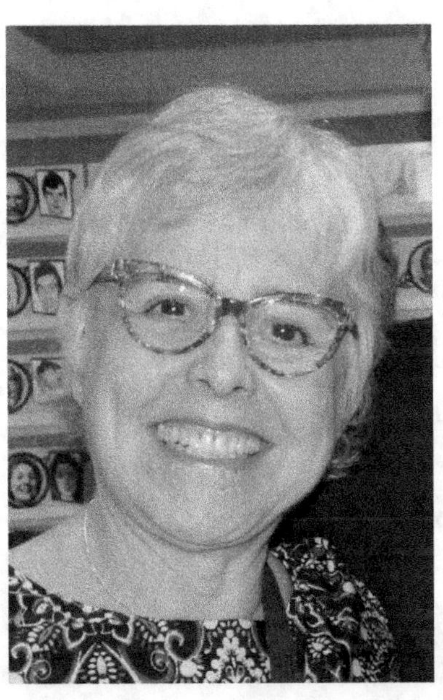

Oh, when I started my first year of med school in the seventies, computers were mainframes and had just arrived at the university. What was that unfamiliar machine, what could I do with it? I started learning a programming language and became an intern at the computer center. I fell in love with the technology because I realized I could do much more with it. Instead of being a physician for one person, I could affect the lives of many, many people. I was very much into decision support systems, the beginning of artificial intelligence expert systems, and so on.

My intention was to provide decision support systems at the point of care. That's what drove me to health informatics and to do a doctorate and my thesis on decision support systems. It was hard for women to be involved in science, technology, engineering, and math, and it still is today. My graduating class was record-breaking: 52 percent of the students were female.

I hear medical school has become a "feminine" profession. They say it's because physicians don't make more money. Yeah, that's true. It was not so hard. And I never felt it was a problem because I was a woman. We were a group of five and we used to work overnight doing last debugging of our systems. It was really fun.

2. After the pandemic is brought under control, what changes do you expect to see appearing in healthcare?

Before the pandemic, teleconsultations were not allowed. Now they are live, and a huge number of teleconsultations are happening all over Brazil. Telemedicine is here to stay and will continually evolve. That's the first thing. The other is providing information necessary to make better decisions. Never in history has information been so necessary. How many ICU beds are occupied? How many ventilators, and where are they? How do I distribute them? So, the need for the whole network of logistics, and deploying and collecting data at the point of care, and interoperability between the different parts of the healthcare network. That is a problem in my country, and I guess in your country as well. Regional health networks are organized around the big technology vendors, like Cerner or Epic, but we need those networks to share information.

So, the issue of sharing information, connecting the different dots of the healthcare network, is essential as we evolve for the future era, and future pandemics. Interoperability for me is a key issue for information-sharing.

3. What do you think are the most significant problems facing professionals working in healthcare?

Always the lack of information at the point of care. With proper decision support, at least you can see a patient in the hospital and you get an idea what's happened before. We need interoperability; we need those standards to do our work. I am very hopeful everybody is going towards that direction. We have the national patient summary. I think the IPS initiative is a very good one.

4. What are the top three reasons you continue to work in health-care, and how might that change in the next two, five, or ten years?

Creating much more quality above all, and much more safety. I believe cost is also an issue, but not the most important one. I would say it's quality and safety. So, for the next two years, I think we'll still see only the strands of interoperability. Telehealth, telemonitoring data, data analytics, data lakes, and so on will evolve as we move ahead. It's very difficult because technology evolves very, very fast, but this time we'll have intelligent companions, maybe robots, to help us. I don't believe they will replace physicians, but they might allow us to have more compassion, to remember what it was to be a medical doctor many, many years ago. Because soon we will have the tools that will provide us with the information we need at the point of care.

And of course the patient engagement. I think we are not good at that. I think some countries are doing fantastic work, like in Slovenia; NHS is strong in England. There are interesting, mobile app solutions that engage patients. I think we really have to engage the patient in their treatment.

5. How would you suggest improving and reforming healthcare?

I think universal care is essential and everybody has to have that right; proper and affordable healthcare. It need not be completely free, but it must be affordable. In many countries it is not so universal. I believe you must work hard on primary care, because if you increase investment in primary care, you wouldn't have so many complications of diabetes, hypertension, and so on. I really am very fond of the Brazilian family health program. It has proven that we can decrease infant mortality and modern mortality. We can decrease hospitalizations for strokes and so on. When we have to go to the patient's home, we must insure they are taking the proper medicine. We need to invest more in primary care and also interoperability, for the information exchange between all in the healthcare network.

I think that is the key issue. And that is the challenge for all of us, because we still don't have that basic foundation.

Chapter 2

Healthcare IT: The Digital Conundrum

"To be, or not to be: that is the question:
Whether 'tis nobler in the mind to suffer
The slings and arrows of outrageous fortune,
Or to take arms against a sea of troubles,
And by opposing end them."
—William Shakespeare, *Hamlet*, Act III, Scene I

At the close of Chapter 1, the subjects of change and adaptation were introduced. During the outbreak of the COVID-19 pandemic in early 2020, a phrase often seen or heard in the media was "the new normal." If there is a new normal, it is one fraught with change and demanding our adaptation. What was normal, and what is normal now? Were our work and our lives in healthcare normal before the pandemic? Is that the normal we would wish to return to?

As human beings, we desire a semblance of predictable normalcy in our lives. However, the World Health Organization (WHO) has advised that the COVID-19 strain of the coronavirus may join other viruses that have come and not gone away, such as SARS or HIV or the Spanish, Asian, and Hong Kong influenzas.

Perhaps both epidemics and pandemics are becoming yet another new normal. If so, we cannot allow ourselves to be caught flat-footed as we were in 2020.

The term "new normal" becomes Hamlet's metaphorical sword of Damocles: Shall we allow ourselves to suffer from this and other misfortunes of humanity (World War II comes to mind), or do we choose to fight and drive them from our lives? Clearly, this is not a simple challenge for healthcare. We cannot issue a recall like an auto manufacturer or text customers an app update, as would a software company. When it comes to having or treating illness, we often find ourselves faced with that Damoclean danger. Perhaps we always will. Perhaps we can change that dynamic.

We clinicians feel a powerful, deeply compelling need to treat and heal our patients. That is our job. COVID-19 has caused, and will continue to wreak, immense harm on the entire world population, but also to ourselves and our own healthcare workers: doctors, nurses, nursing home workers, EMTs. While it raged we were all at risk, and many suffered from depression, anxiety, insomnia, and the profound fear of contracting the virus, then transmitting it to our family and others close to us. Some died. None of this is going away—perhaps mitigating to some extent but perhaps never. A pandemic of this order conveys the dread and fear that exude from terrorism attacks: we do not know if or when we are going to be the next to fall ill or even perhaps die. That is no way to live.

Yes, there are COVID-19 vaccines, and they will work, but how well? For how long? For how many different types of individuals? If vaccines work now, will we discover better alternatives a year from now? Will the vaccine's immunity wane, and when will we need a booster? Will the virus mutate, making the current vaccines ineffective, requiring new vaccines and vaccination efforts? Even more important, how do we adapt to a new normal in which we are never immune to viral attacks? Can we, at least, have a shared agreement of beliefs and practices in our healthcare systems? Cannot we work together to fashion a redesigned, data-driven system so that we can take on the next pressing health matter—whether it is climate change or alcoholism or adolescent obesity or even another pandemic—in stride? Should not this be our overarching goal?

It is quite clear that this approach thus far—by which I mean piling on little changes going back at least a century, to the great influenza virus of 1918—has not worked well. We continually try to tamp out diseases—for example, influenza, diabetes, the common cold, hypertension. If this is in fact the new normal in healthcare, is it a desirable new normal? Of course it is not. If we are to truly embrace this new normal, then let us do so by seeking a systemic remedy for our healthcare processes. Let us use fresh, new problem definitions, with accompanying new possible solutions deployed with powerful technology-based tools and techniques.

Can We Really Fix Healthcare?

Yes. There is a solution, and it is found in healthcare resources and tools we already have. These resources and tools await our taking them up to do battle in our ever-roiling sea of disarray and troubles. Simply put, the solution is to implement a more significant role for healthcare information technology. This is not the old IT you might be thinking of, but a "new normal" version I have named *revolutionary healthcare information technology.*

John Gantz, senior vice president at International Data Corporation (IDC), says, "It's been a long time since the IT organization reported to the facilities management department in many hospitals, yet they should. IT's digital processes need to cohere with the hospital's, regardless if they are analog, digital, or sneakers. Healthcare providers traditionally have lagged other industries in adopting the latest IT technologies and IT processes. They need to be on the forefront of balancing the stability of their organization—in other words, running the business effectively—with the vitality that enables innovation and improvement. Some of this is IT's fault for not asking for what it needs and allowing capital acquisitions to be decided upon by functional departments. And there is more data, information, and knowledge than any single entity can reasonably be expected to analyze and benefit from. IT can take a leadership role, not simply in assessing technology acquisitions, but in showing how to derive more value from the data pouring from the cornucopia."

But the greater impact is much more human-centered. HIT is often not considered an equal partner at the table when the senior management committee is working on issues and solving problems. I think it is safe to assume that few if any colleagues stop by their CIO's office and ask, "What can we do about the COVID-19 pandemic?" or "We are short-staffed and have a six-hour wait list in the ED for non-life-threatening illnesses. How can you help?"

Revolutionary HIT can help by leveraging existing data to further optimize processes—that is, if there are intelligent, optimized processes in place. They must be designed, not by default, but rather intelligently conceived. Administrators, clinicians, and HIT management must work together to design them. This is the new normal: enabling "smart" healthcare management to streamline the workflow and help improve access to care and use of limited resources. Allowing clinicians to assure high-quality care is being dispensed so that patients are having exceptional experiences and health outcomes. All the necessary data is already in your organization's repository, waiting to be used. HIT has an enlightened, professional staff, waiting to study that data and help make forward-looking decisions about its use. Your people want to perform as many elective surgeries, diagnostic images, therapeutic treatments, and routine checkups as there are patients needing them.

Administrative management wants to stay on top of unusually high costs that can be intelligently reduced, billing and reimbursements, complex scheduling, the supply chain, and HR resourcing challenges to expand care delivery, improve clinical outcomes, and bolster revenues. All these aspects of healthcare delivery can be digitally integrated by revolutionary HIT into an interoperable system that automates the workflow for maximum efficiency and measurable financial performance.

Bedside Consult: A Brief History of Computers in Healthcare

In the 1950s, computers were mammoth machines, rightly thought to provide utilitarian service like the electric company or the public water and sewer works. Today, computer technology is embedded in practically every device we use. It will come as no surprise to learn that computers were born of calculators and so early business uses were focused on managing numbers: accounting. Their use in healthcare was no exception. But over time, computers were taught to process transactions and by the late 1950s to store large quantities of data, then use it in differing situations, for instance interfacing inventory management with purchasing.

By the mid-1950s, however, the study of informatics was launched, beginning in healthcare and eventually spreading to other areas of application. Informatics, a term often favored by academics, has become something of a catchall euphemism altogether similar to computer science. The American Medical Informatics Association defines it: "Biomedical and health informatics applies principles of computer and information science to the advancement of life sciences research, health professions education, public health, and patient care. This multidisciplinary and integrative field focuses on health information technologies (HIT), and involves the computer, cognitive, and social sciences."

In the 1960s, the need to provide patient data to Medicare and Medicaid drove an influx in computer use, and a few vendors began designing computer systems for healthcare. However, the sword of Damocles defined that moment: healthcare did not understand how to use computers, and computer vendors did not understand how to design computer systems for healthcare. Nevertheless, the focus widened to include processing patient personal information, diagnoses, and care plans.

In 1969, Dr. Lawrence Weed, at the University Medical Center in Burlington, VT, developed PROMIS, the Problem Oriented Medical Information System, which integrated every aspect of healthcare, from front-office administration to procedure and laboratory test fees to patient treatment. PROMIS "did not have wide acceptance. To accept it meant a change in the power structure, something that did not begin to happen until the 1990s when the advent of managed care in the U.S. in all its variations reinvigorated a push towards patient-centered information systems."

In the mid-1970s, computer use in healthcare became a focus of interest. Learning to use and operate them was a task assigned to nurses. Doctors continued to scribble abbreviated notes on paper for someone else to decipher and input. Meanwhile, the EHR was introduced in 1972 by the Regenstrief Institute of Indianapolis. Later in that decade, SUMEX, the Stanford University Medical Experimental computer resource, implemented an online data communications technology, facilitating access to electronic databases for information sharing, and second diagnostic opinions from external sources.

In 1980, Dr. Edward Shortliffe founded the first program of study in biomedical informatics at Stanford University. Earlier, he created MYCIN, an AI-based expert system that identified bacteria causing severe infections and suggested antibiotics with which to treat them.

The 1980s also saw the introduction of CADUCEUS, an AI-infused medical diagnosis system developed by University of Pittsburgh professor Harry Pople, from years of interviews with Dr. Jack Meyers. CADUCEUS could diagnose over one thousand diseases and was able to pass an internal medicine board examination.

Clive Finkelstein rocked the IT world in 1980 with his new concept, information engineering. Finkelstein's emphasis on information engineering was, to use the title of Stephen Greenblatt's book, a startling swerve from the prevailing data-collection mindset. Computers could be used to turn data into information with which to make informed decisions. Engineered information had greater value because it could be modeled, remodeled, taken apart, and reassembled in different configurations. In a word, thusly engineered computer-based information could be used to extract highly informed and valuable knowledge. The relationship is often characterized graphically as layers, or a pyramid, and referred to as the DIKW hierarchy, this way:

- Data

- Information

- Knowledge

- Wisdom

James Martin, the famed technology futurist and author of over one hundred books, including the bestselling *The Wired Society*, observed in the 1980s how long it took products of all shapes, colors, and sizes to get to market—often seven to ten years. It was an analog world, and it showed. Martin, among his many accomplishments (as in working with Clive Finkelstein on information engineering), introduced his conception of rapid application development (RAD) for software engineering and forever transformed the task of designing new and updating existing software applications. Martin's RAD, introduced in his eponymous book in 1991, changed the very nature of programming, and thus product development, and in its way spearheaded the waves of entrepreneurial innovation we still see today. The two premises upon which RAD is based are prototyping and developing iterations, and will be discussed again. We were at the tipping point of becoming a digital world.

By the mid-1990s, early handheld computers, termed personal data assistants (PDAs), appeared as managed care proliferated and healthcare became more directed toward patient outcomes. Apple's Newton vied for a role in healthcare, unsuccessfully, yet today the iPhone is widely used.

Meanwhile, today, in the twenty-first century, much attention has focused on the EHR, and its uneven use and lack of standards. HL7 is a standards-setting organization trying to solve the problem, which is seriously exacerbated by the fact that there are over a thousand software solution providers. Fast Healthcare Interoperability Resources (FHIR) is the latest standard holding great promise to address the problem of limited interoperability.

Understanding the Digital Conundrum

The emergence of the digital age in healthcare, which dates back to the mid- to latter years of the twentieth century, was not greeted with joy and accolades, but rather a great deal of skepticism. Similarly, IT found the business and operational aspects of healthcare difficult to serve with its already established business-based products and services, which were a poor fit. All that has changed: the twenty-first century digital revolution has accelerated medical research, patient awareness, and AI-infused everything. There is an entire software industry dedicated to healthcare—yet another sword of Damocles.

Today, there is a healthy harmony and a we-can-do-it attitude between clinical and HIT people, working together to identify and resolve problems. All we have to change is our attitude. Making this essential attitudinal adjustment is at the essence of the relationship between HIT and clinicians. Yes, HIT is a servant of the clinician, helping them make better decisions to achieve better outcomes. Yes, doctors have a level of knowledge unsurpassed. The challenge is to deploy the HIT resources so they fit the clinician's needs and achieve the greatest impact with the least disruption to the clinician and the delivery of clinical care. Just as IT has consistently moved toward working more closely with the core business, so has it also shifted from a confederation of technocrats to a service organization. By adopting a similar shift, HIT can become an instrumental partner in reshaping twenty-first-century healthcare. In so doing, it will find new opportunities, challenges, and successes for its efforts.

Getting HIT Involved

Healthcare IT in most instances is either underperforming or underutilized. It is the equivalent of owning a Ferrari and only driving it at five miles an hour. Our first task is to launch the HIT revolution. As previously stated, the promise of this book is:

> *Revolutionary Healthcare Information Technology* (RHIT) offers clinicians, researchers, and administrators immensely powerful tools to drive clinical and administrative processes to deliver high-quality, safe, accessible, and investment-responsible medical outcomes.

There are so many ways in which HIT could add value to healthcare administration and practice—if only asked to bring its expertise to bear. The IT organization, as it has proven in thousands of other industries and enterprises, is masterful at developing systematic approaches to solving problems.

Today's healthcare organization operates in crisis mode nearly all the time. Everyone is overworked. Caregivers race from one emergency to the next, all too accurately portrayed on *Grey's Anatomy*. Healthcare's intelligent processes, where they actually exist, are shunted aside for a variety of disingenuous reasons. Where to start fixing things?

So What Is the Problem?

The problem is with workflow. Healthcare's workflows are not well defined to provide the desired outcomes. They are variable, ever-changing, inefficient, and poorly integrated with the patient's journey. HIT can be of immense value in designing and implementing a "new-normal" systematic construct for the delivery of services and the management of healthcare. Like the Corps of Engineers getting a river back into its banks, it is what they do.

In order to establish a realistic and productive workflow, the first two matters that need immediate attention are the EHR and interoperability. Since its inception on paper and a clipboard, the patient record has represented the headwaters, the first and foremost repository of patient information. While providing a digital repository, EHR vendors sidestepped on their responsibilities for creating tools that delivered better outcomes. For example, they never prioritized complete interoperability. Instead, they concentrated on the easy task of recordkeeping and took a pass on clinical operations. As providers, the government, and software vendors squabbled over standards and contested implementation best practices, it became a fundamental digital conundrum. This is especially true of healthcare organizations where different practices and functions use different EHRs. Exchanging the data among the EHR records inhibits a manageable workflow for patient care. The result is a diminished patient experience and suboptimal outcomes. It is a problem that can be resolved with help from revolutionary HIT. Its solution will go far toward the healthcare environment becoming more efficient and progressive.

Simply stated, interoperability is unifying all the divergent computer systems and applications so they can, in IT parlance, "talk to one another." In the 1970s, systems were designed for billing and claims, not patient care. Few saw a need for interoperability in those times. With the advent of the single-sourced EHR in the 1990s, interoperability became critical and complex to implement. Even so, we have made progress: client-server to networks to the internet to cloud computing have established common platforms for hardware interoperability, but certain software apps still pose challenges. Vendors must shoulder some of the blame for the lack of interoperability today; as with EHRs, each wants to preserve its competitive advantage by making it difficult for healthcare organizations to switch to another vendor. Again, we must ask for revolutionary HIT to help resolve this problem, both in our current operations and into the foreseeable future.

All these computer issues and problems set clinicians on edge, which bleeds into their perceptions of HIT in general. The more HIT can step in and lend a hand, the sooner better solutions can be reached. But as suggested earlier, it is all about attitude. So let us step back a few paces and, in the next chapter, examine how we can create and manage the change and adaptation necessary to revolutionize healthcare.

The RHIT Interview: Gareth Sherlock, Chief Information Officer, Cleveland Clinic, London, England

1. What was the most significant event or factor that determined your pursuing a career in healthcare?

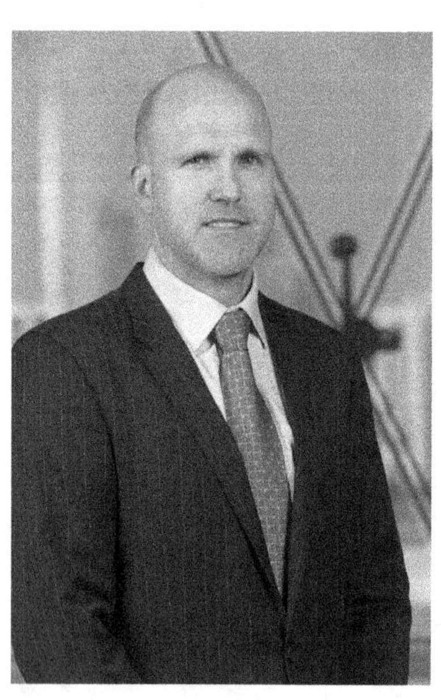

I graduated from Sydney University with a Chemical Engineering degree (Honors), as well as a degree in Finance. I started my career working for about ten months as a chemical engineer and quickly realized I was not going to make a very good engineer. I decided to make a big career change and took a job with Anderson Consulting (now Accenture) as a Technology Consultant. It was a fantastic graduate program and I really enjoyed the work; the whole creative career path and the way they developed you. I started off in the finance industry, but then transitioned on to a healthcare project, implementing a clinical information system across eight metropolitan hospitals and fourteen renal facilities in the state of South Australia. My brother was an orthopedic surgeon, so I thought, why not give healthcare a try. I worked on the project for three years.

I loved the work I did and I love the healthcare industry. I became very passionate about staying in healthcare. I did about eleven years of healthcare consulting with Accenture in Australia, the UK, and across Europe. Then I started a project in Abu Dhabi with Cleveland Clinic, helping build a new 365-bed multi-specialty hospital. That's where I transitioned from consulting to working with a provider. I've been with the clinic for the last eleven years and after Abu Dhabi, I moved with the Cleveland Clinic, again helping to open a 185-bed multi-specialty hospital in central London.

So that was how I fell into healthcare—and I've been there ever since and love it.

2. After the pandemic is brought under control, what changes do you expect to see appearing in healthcare?

Healthcare hasn't really changed at its core. Our mission is still helping patients get access to the care they need, with a focus around the patient experience and caregiver experience. There has, however, been a big shift in areas like virtual health and remote care. Will healthcare organizations be able to maintain the gains they've made in virtual care?

It feels like we have made five years of gain in the space of a few months. But as the lockdowns are lifted, many of the gains made in virtual care have disappeared. It's important that we don't lose sight of how effective healthcare organizations have become since transitioning to virtual systems. We need to build more virtual and remote care into traditional care pathways. This can significantly improve both the patient and caregiver experience.

Another new trend is hybrid staffing models. A lot of nonclinical staff have moved very quickly to remote work, and many of these roles will not return to the office. The whole office dynamic has also changed because of the pandemic, and organizations are adapting very quickly to this new normal.

3. What do you think are the most significant problems facing professionals working in healthcare?

Many of the big problems in healthcare are the same as before COVID, but some have been amplified by it. For example, caregiver burnout for clinicians and physicians has become more of an issue.

Nurses are really challenged because of the prolonged intensity of this pandemic. Technology needs to continue playing a big role in improving the caregiver experience. We need to implement technology to make the caregivers' lives better. Caregivers need to spend less time in front of a computer and more time taking care of patients. Organizations focusing on this are also going to attract the best caregivers.

Patients also want to be more empowered. Healthcare needs to continue looking at other industries to understand how to improve the patient experience.

4. What are the top three reasons you continue to work in healthcare, and how might that change in the next two, five, or ten years?

That's a great question. I've never wanted to leave healthcare because I feel it's the most rewarding industry to work in. You are helping to change people's lives, as well as helping people get access to the care they need. Maybe there's no better industry to work in and nothing more rewarding. The people working in the industry are also just brilliant. I really enjoy coming to work every day because of the people I work with, and the people I get to meet.

5. How would you suggest improving and reforming healthcare?

I think one of the biggest issues we need to solve in healthcare globally is access. We need to make it a priority in healthcare for people to easily access the care they need.

In the UK, we have the NHS, which is a great system that the country is very proud of. What other country would have a fifteen-minute tribute to their health system at the opening ceremony of the Olympic Games? The NHS does, however, have access challenges with long waiting lists. In other countries without public health systems as comprehensive as the NHS, there are access issues of a different kind. This is not an easy problem to solve, but it is something we need to figure out globally.

CHAPTER 3

The Management of Change

"In my opinion, the pandemic was not a question of if. It was a question of when. And I think virtually all of my colleagues agree there will be another pandemic virus. My question is, are we going to learn the critical and painful lessons that we've learned from this one, and are we going to be able to apply that knowledge to the next pandemic so that fewer people die?"

—Angela Rasmussen, PhD virologist at VIDO-InterVac, a research institute at the University of Saskatchewan

A healthcare research report published in 2012 stated, "As hospitals focus on cost control and the need to deliver high-quality care, their challenge has never been greater to meet the needs of their community and ensure long-term financial sustainability, even as reimbursements and budgets are ratcheted down."

Almost ten years on, it seems fair to ask, "What's new?" Sadly, as insightful as this statement is, healthcare can do no more than pay lip service to it. Even more distressing, this concern dates back much, much further. No other industry—not an automaker, an oil patch producer, a retailer—would survive if it overlooked this simple challenge.

It seems evident to the reflective healthcare professional that, built into these perennial challenges facing healthcare, is our issue with change. Change happens all the time, to all of us. But that means change is in control, and leaves us to react to it. The changes in healthcare we need to implement are proactive, chosen, and made of our own volition. The essential tools for asserting our control are digital, and they are available from our own revolutionary HIT organization.

The front-page headline in the *New York Times* on May 24, 2020, read:

U.S. Deaths Near 100,000, An Incalculable Loss

Of course deaths have skyrocketed since then, not only in the United States but globally. Clearly, a proactive, forward-thinking healthcare enterprise would never have knowingly promulgated a headline such as this. Yet here we are, still fighting the scourge in reactive mode. Are we fulfilling the tenets of the Hippocratic Oath? If not, why are these goals so difficult to achieve? Perhaps it is as simple as Dr. M. Scott Peck, wrote: "Human beings are poor examiners, subject to superstition, bias, prejudice, and a PROFOUND tendency to see what they want to see rather than what is really there."

In 2020, a shocking realization hit U.S. healthcare: they were unprepared to deal with a pandemic in so many ways—staffing, supplies, funds, profitable business lines, high-quality care lines to remain competitive, just to name a few. To survive, provider organizations learned they had to quickly restore their non-critical revenue streams while preparing for the anticipated multiple waves of the COVID-19 pandemic. Successful recovery for these organizations would not be represented by a return to the former ways: the business was no longer viable. As suggested by the catchphrase "the new normal," everything would be changing, whether anyone liked it or not. The road to recovery would require phased responses to myriad challenges that lay ahead. It was a new way of thinking about healthcare delivery. Everyone would have to contribute to creating a more nimble and responsive organization that could deliver better outcomes and streamlined patient experiences.

Bedside Consult: Open Notes, a Change Management Tool

Not very many years ago, a college student had no way to give a professor or a course their feedback. Then along came a website, Rate My Professors, and everything changed. Thanks to internet technology, students could share their thoughts with their teachers, the college administration, and other students. Needless to say, educators balked and fussed over this change, but in time came to realize https://www.ratemyprofessors.com was a powerful change management tool.

Healthcare has been similarly resistant to patient feedback. Yet today we have the Open Notes program, an initiative launched by Beth Israel Deaconess Medical Center (affiliated with Harvard Medical School).

Open Notes led Beth Israel to support another program called OurNotes, where the patient initiates a history of present illnesses (HPI) and their own personal health goals. Its use has expanded to telehealth. Clinicians sharing their notes found that workloads were not significantly changed, and most felt sharing notes led to a better relationship with their patients. Many have found that the fact their notes would be read by others led them to improving the organization, expression, and information they were documenting, resulting in the creation of best practices in note-writing. Between

75 and 85 percent of patients queried in one study said having access to their clinicians' notes made them feel a more confident sense of participation in their healthcare.

Another progressive change is set to take effect in April 2021, called the Cures Act Final Rule from the U.S. Department of Health and Human Services' (HHS) Office of the National Coordinator for Health IT (ONC). It was released with final notations regarding the information blocking provision and adopted new HIT certification requirements that make smartphone access to health information available at no cost. Dr. Don Rucker (interviewed elsewhere in these pages), has stated that through the use of application programming interfaces (APIs), ONC found "strong support for advancing patient access and clinician coordination through the provisions in the final rule. We look forward to continuing to work with everyone to get patients the benefits of modern technology that they have not had to date in healthcare, though they've had that in every other part of their lives."

Rucker credits COVID-19 for some of the innovations we have seen in healthcare since its onset. Telehealth is certainly a big one, but so is the Cares Act, which began life in 2009—over twelve years ago.

What We Think about When We Think about Change

When most people think about change, their attitude varies from sighs to resignation to resistance. Change is rarely viewed as something positive; we tend not to look forward to its influences. Yet with change being a constant in all human experience and behavior, why is this so? Why do we resist change? Why do we prefer to think we are comfortable with things just as they are? We do not want to rock the boat. We do not want to fix things we do not think are broken. And the last thing we want to do is actively promote and drive—manage—change. Change management is a task better left to someone else. At some later time, we might decide whether or not we want to get on board with it. Perhaps we use the excuse that it is above our pay grade.

Principles of change. For the purposes of our discussion, here is how I view change.

1. Change is inevitable. We have the choice to either allow random, unpredictable change or to manage change to the best of our ability.

2. Change is not inherently dissociative or bad. It has no connotations of goodness or evil. Einstein said the measure of intelligence is in one's capacity for change. Winston Churchill said, "To improve is to change; to be perfect is to change often."

3. There are two types of change that the healthcare worker confronts on a daily basis: immediate, disruptive change, and gradual, insistent change.

Disruptive change is like working in the ED—you never know what the next patient's problem will be: a heart attack, an auto accident, a stroke.

Insistent change builds up gradually, like seeing a trend line documenting an increase in specific chronic disease visiting a clinic or the rise in the use of a particular addictive pain medication.

Both types of change have the effect of being either positive or negative influences in the way they affect the healthcare facility. Disruptive change usually cannot be accounted for; its basic nature is random. But insistent change can be more orderly, even process-driven, which is proven by tracking Kondratieff cycles. COVID-19 is certainly an example of a disruptive change that turned into insistent change. Either type of change may begin as positive or negative, but some often do a one-eighty turn and become the other. I term these changepoints.

> A *changepoint* is a significant moment of recognition that something is not the way it ought to be, or perhaps is not the way it has always been in the past. Now it is uncommon and remarkable. Some changepoints, more often the insistent than the disruptive type, can be anticipated with Kondratieff cycles, which means they can be studied with digital databases and statistical analysis tools. Pasteur's accidental discovery of penicillin was just such a disruptive changepoint; he had not been studying mold on bread for this purpose. COVID-19 was expected, but it was not properly anticipated, for myriad reasons it is this book's intention to address and help correct.

As David Bowie said in his eponymous song about change, all we do is turn and face one strange change after another. For at least the past forty years, healthcare has been whipsawed by both external and internal change. Most of these changes are rent upon healthcare. They are changes healthcare had not chosen for itself and resists—in other words, healthcare has gone into a defensive stance. By using changepoints to identify and diagnostically chart change, it is possible for revolutionary healthcare to go on the offensive, choosing the change it perceives a need for and pushing back against changes driven by random and uncontrollable forces.

Because we deal with illness and unhealthy people, it may seem natural that we have a dour outlook. It does not need to be that way. We tend to focus on our prescribed daily details and routines, without allowing much time or thought given over to how things are working or how they might be improved upon. Yet the work we do is intended to heal the sick, and that should be the focus of all our work efforts because restoring health is positive change and the most sought-after outcome. If we are not achieving this, consistently and at a very high success ratio, we need to examine what needs to change so we can improve our outcomes.

Managed by Change or the Management of Change?

Change is running the show for healthcare management and us, its diverse workforce, on its terms instead of ours, spreading disruptive and harmful disease. We need look no further than the disruptive change caused by COVID-19 to see this on a massive scale. But insistent change can also have detrimental effects: administration that is inundated with more and more disparate data, either from the cloud, the computer, or on paper, than it can assimilate; workflows that do not deliver quality care at an affordable cost; a chronic shortage of clinicians—the list is endless and ever-changing.

Peter F. Drucker, regarded as the father of modern management, was so concerned about managing change that he wrote one of his thirty-nine books about it, *Managing in a Time of Great Change*. Drucker believed that the most effective way to manage change is to create it—another way of saying to go on the offensive. Permitting change to be in charge means letting go of control and allowing chaos to reign. Instead of letting change manage us, we need to take control of, and manage, change ourselves—both individually and collectively. This applies to absolutely everyone in the healthcare organization: the cleaning crews, valets, clerical workers, pharma workers, clinicians, nurses, the doctors. Everyone can provide meaningful input for managing change.

Strategy. Where to begin? The first critical success practice for creating positive change—change we can be in charge of—is having a strategy. Simply defined, a strategy is how you achieve your intended objective. Of course, you must first have that objective. Many doctors' offices and hospitals have a mission statement; that is their objective. If you do not have one, or need to reevaluate the one you do have, this proven model for defining strategy has four parts:

1. Formulating a plan

2. Organizing the resources for executing the plan

3. Guiding and moving the plan into action, and

4. Controlling the variables that crop up so that you achieve your goal.

While there are many computer-based tools and techniques for strategizing, this one can be created with discussion, pen, and paper.

Drucker spoke of having a thorough understanding of the business—in our case, the healthcare enterprise—as essential to implementing a strategy for change. He defined this understanding as assumptions, but today we might better refer to them as business model building blocks:

- What is the economic and business environment, and your healthcare facility's mission and its core competencies?

- All three building blocks must harmoniously integrate with one another.

- Everyone must understand the first three blocks, and work for their achievement.

- These blocks must be constantly challenged and regularly reaffirmed to achieve the necessary competencies and successful outcomes.

Establishing these building blocks and obtaining buy-in from every employee is not simple, nor will it happen overnight. Most organizations, in attempting to create an agreement and understanding of this kind, meet in groups for months, even years at times. Goals and progress points are essential. A means of creating this business model and the management of change that accompanies it will be elaborated on more in Chapter 4.

Interestingly, Drucker could have been discussing interoperability. As discussed in Chapter 2, EHRs and interoperability present the gateway to forward-looking healthcare strategy and change. This, of course, cannot be achieved without buy-in from all stakeholders and the full participation of HIT. In the same way there are few, if any, practical ways to create interoperability between, say, a shoe store, ice cream shop, and an interior design store in a shopping mall, healthcare must develop and deploy a holistic strategy that incorporates interoperability to support its disparate processes. Consider that the country doctor a hundred or more years ago was expected to do anything the patient needed. Specialized medical care has grown and developed into numerous sub-specialties—for example orthopedics, cardiology, neurology, pediatrics—which became a way to enhance market share and enhance outcomes. In most cases, they were designed as discrete silos of medicine, using old business development tools, each as a distinct, stand-alone care stream. Our objective is to evolve the global healthcare system into a twenty-first-century model of how healthcare ought to be, not to continue with how it operated for over a hundred years in the past. By de-siloing or combining some of these processes, they can be oriented into primary, trackable, precisely defined, and far more productive and economical workflows, which could be implemented with the assistance of revolutionary HIT. That is an important aspect of achieving interoperability.

All together now. This is the most important changepoint that needs to be addressed in our profession. Connective, systemic, interoperable healthcare information technology is the transformative solution to managing this fragmentation. It is utterly unimaginable what will happen to our healthcare system if we fail to improve our systems and processes. The solution and the help we need to do this lie squarely in the deployment of revolutionary HIT.

Through a glass, darkly. We see the healthcare system from the inside, more than likely in the same way as the blind men in the fable about each trying to describe an elephant. If the fragmentation need be any more difficult to understand, we only have to look at the fact that, each year, nearly twenty million American medical tourists go outside the country for care because the U.S. system is up to 70 percent more expensive (which includes administrative costs), while foreign medical tourists come to America for healthcare because they perceive it as the best available anywhere in the world—and can afford it. Medical tourism has driven some domestic healthcare enterprises, anxious to recapture lost revenues, to actually open facilities in other countries. This is yet another unanticipated way we see the absence of cohesion, business planning, and interoperability—and so we have another conundrum.

Solutions, not blame. I hope you have seen that a higher level of structural organization and collaborative purpose is the path to workable, sustainable solutions. We gain nothing by pointing out mistakes and mis-directions. That is the past. We must learn to change and develop new ways of managing our healthcare organization at the highest levels of operational integrity today so that we, and it, have a future. To achieve this requires everyone in the healthcare enterprise participating in a collaborative effort. You, I am sure, have heard of collaboration, a great concept but one to which we usually only pay lip service. Its goals are often unclear, but not in this case. Our collaborative mission is to rescue and resuscitate our livelihood and our mission.

Collaborating with HIT. Revolutionary HIT will help drive the change essential to restoring our healthcare system as the leading edge of medical innovation. But first, healthcare needs a plan. This is a job for administrators, clinicians, partners, and policy-shapers, to work together with HIT in order to manage essential change, both for the short- and the long-term value proposition. HIT has the means of transforming clinics and hospitals, helping to bring about the essential change that must occur in healthcare delivery. COVID-19 has shut down or forced the acquisitions of hundreds of hospitals in the U.S. that were caught unprepared in so many ways. Some learned the hard way they were uncompetitive in the marketplace and lacked the organizational resources to deal with the pandemic. COVID-19 has also driven thousands of doctors and nurses out of the medical profession. Efficient, progressive change management works, as has been proven over and over in other business enterprises. It must be better applied in healthcare.

Clinical and administrative processes impact patient outcomes, and therefore impact costs of doing business from admission to discharge. In addition, doctors and nurses are reluctant to give up control over their processes and are disinterested in financial balance sheets. They argue, "We always did it this way, so why should we change?" or "But my patients are different." It is hard to change this mindset, but it must change if there is to be any hope of changing processes. Those who undertake this challenge must possess a deep knowledge of the clinical setting, the clinician's buy-in, an understanding of workflow principles, and, last but far from least, an information technology grounding. When confronted with Hydra-headed problems such as these, aerospace companies often held secret, off-site meetings, attended by a select few, to solve the problem. They called these legendary meetings "skunk works."

The uses for computer technology are limited only by our imagination, determining the new application for the task, and then, perhaps most important, strategizing how to get the job done. Much like our brain's abilities, most information technology resources, irrespective of their uses or application in a given enterprise, are underutilized. I believe revolutionary technology can pave the way to get HIT working harder for both healthcare administrators and clinicians. Revolutionary HIT has the means to address that underutilized aspect of technology and put it to work for the healthcare organization.

Neither healthcare workers nor most patients wish to see "the new normal" return to the normal of yesteryear. It is also quite possible that they see the tasks involved in building a changepoint-based enterprise as being someone else's job. It is not. Everyone needs to pitch in, accept, and drive change for creating a new, most excellent healthcare organization. We must regain the public's trust in our competencies, because we are the most important industry in the world. If the public loses trust, our social fabric frays, tears, and is destroyed.

Think about how you would transform your organization into the "new normal." Bear in mind that change is neither good nor bad, but thinking makes it so. Keep notes on what you would consider changepoints, and discuss them with others. The next chapter provides a way to carry these thoughts into actions.

The RHIT Interview: Thomas M. Koulopoulos, president and founder of the Delphi Group think tank and author of *Reimagining Healthcare*, Boston, Massachusetts

1. What was the most significant event or factor that determined your pursuing a career in technology?

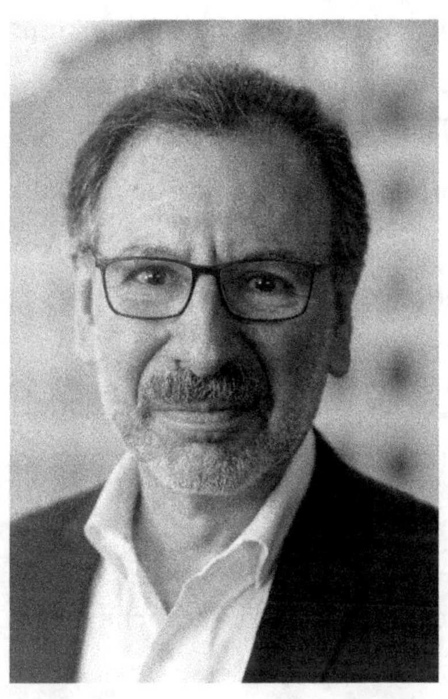

I grew up with a father who was an engineer. Everything turned into a life lesson on how things work. On weekends, when most fathers took their kids to Little League or a sporting event, my dad took me to Radio Shack. So I can't even remember a time when I wasn't into technology. In college, I thought I'd get into business. I struggled in all my business courses, but aced programming languages and relational databases. That's when I had a kind of awakening: that this must be what I'm meant to do. It was all about the latest tech. I loved it, lived it—and I still do.

For me, technology is fun. There's no problem that can't be solved with the right technologies.

2. After the pandemic is brought under control, what changes do you expect to see appearing in healthcare?

Here are three from my observations.

One, the simplest changes, but maybe the most profound, will be our transition to telehealth and telemedicine. I think people are starting to realize virtual office visits can be even more effective than in-person office visits. So much of healthcare is built around [a pre-sumed] convenience for the doctors and an inconvenience for pa-tients. Telehealth helps both. Patient outcomes will improve because we'll use more healthcare. Managing a larger workload through telehealth is much easier and will lead to improved outcomes.

Two, we've got to change our social perspective. The pandemic has created a much higher awareness of clinicians' commitment to helping patients. They are incredibly dedicated to their profession. Recognizing this helps to end the misplaced blame for systemic prob-lems with our process—problems which are not fundamentally the fault of clinicians or healthcare providers. A change in social senti-ment towards clinicians, I think, is a very important part of what we will take away from the COVID experience.

And number three, coming to terms with comorbidities. COVID caused us to realize that as we get older we have multiple condi-tions, each one of which can be critically important in determining our health and quality of life. As we age, we become more suscepti-ble to comorbidities. Unfortunately, COVID is a taste of what health-care will be like when the majority of the population reaches their seventies and eighties.

3. What do you think are the most significant problems facing pro-fessionals working in healthcare?

Workload. Everyone I've spoken with says the same thing: the workload is just immense. So what does that look like? It's not spend-ing the majority of time with the patient, but on administrative work instead. Some of those administrative tasks must be done by clini-cians, but not most of them. They are chores and tasks which should be given to someone more qualified, better skilled, and with the time to do them.

4. What are the top three reasons you continue to work in health-care, and how might that change in the next two, five, or ten years?

Every healthcare worker I have spoken with repeated the same refrain: they got into healthcare because of a deeply rooted desire to help people and alleviate suffering. The drivers behind that are many, but the sentiment is universal. The other two reasons I often hear, hand in hand with the first, are the desire to solve hard problems and the intellectual challenge that entails. Unfortunately, most clinicians end up stuck in an administrative quagmire that makes achieving those objectives incredibly challenging. My hope, and my belief, is that we will see technologies such as AI and machine learning become central to helping alleviate the administrative burden on clinicians. This will allow them to do more of what they are best at, caring for patients and managing complex healthcare issues.

5. How would you suggest improving and reforming healthcare? Maybe you want to write a book about that?

Yes, I wrote a book about healthcare. It's funny; I gave my PCP a copy. He was one of three people I dedicated the book to. He said, "You know, I really hope this book helps fix healthcare." I replied, "You know what? 'Fixing' is the wrong word."

It's a very complex system. There are parts that will continue to be broken because we don't have the ability to take it apart, disman-tle it, put in new parts, and put it back together from scratch. We're maintaining the engines while the plane is in flight, if you will. So I'll settle for something less broken and make small but intentional strides forward. And number one among those is, alleviating the adminis-trative workload for healthcare providers. Number two, increasing access for patients, which I think is absolutely critical. And number three, make the patient experience more pleasant. In other words, treat patients like consumers, with transparency and tools to better coordinate their healthcare as it gets more complex. All of that will inevitably create better outcomes.

Chapter 4

A CAT Scan of Today's Healthcare Business

"Humans have survived as a species, not because we have physical advantages like size, strength, or speed, but because of our ability to connect in social groups. We exchange ideas. We coordinate goals. We share information and emotions."

—Vivek Murthy, MD, Surgeon General and author of *Together*

Legendary business consultant and Harvard Business School professor Michael Porter and I share a love of sports, in particular the competitive, strategic aspects of sports. Since we both live in Boston, we can follow very successful teams in baseball, hockey, basketball, and football. Porter's wisdom was established with his first book, *Competitive Advantage,* in 1985. Healthcare does not have to struggle against the same kind of competition as a business such as Burger King, Costco, or Volkswagen, but nevertheless can learn valuable lessons from how competitive business environments work. Ever the progressive thinker, Porter wrote another seminal book in 2006, *Redefining Health Care: Creating Value-Based Competition on*

Results. Even after fifteen-plus years, its ideas and insights merit a close reading. Why? Because the issues and problems Porter raised with healthcare are the same as those we struggle with today. And today Porter remains a voice in healthcare to be listened to.

- There is no clear set of standards for best practices.

- There are profound imbalances in care, within institutions, in payer compensation, and in demographics and geographics.

- Costs are too high and rising, and do not correlate with quality of care.

- Clinicians are resistant to change and innovation, even in the face of the rising toll of treatment errors and burnout.

Indeed, how is such a state of affairs even remotely possible? Almost any other business would be addressing and correcting these issues as part of its business processes, or competition would weed them out. It would not take a bankruptcy or a natural disaster to spur action. Yet for healthcare, it took a pandemic for it to sit up and pay attention.

What have we learned about our work, our industry, and ourselves from the pandemic? Each of us needs to think very hard about our answers to each of those three questions. Why? Because the heart of the matter is, the answers we provide are those that will assure that our industry thrives and makes up for the missteps, oversights, faulty assumptions, and mistakes it has made in the past. An old saw goes, "Everybody complains about the weather, but no one does anything about it." This typifies how we in healthcare have been regarded for many years, and more importantly, what we must do about improving our profession. We need to start in on a solution today and make things happen. We need to become rainmakers.

Healthcare is a relatively new business entity. It began as an aggregation of different medical and dental services and practitioners, hospitals, clinics, and administrative support services in the early twentieth century.

Before the commercialization of U.S. healthcare and its turn toward a for-profit industry, we had individual doctors and stand-alone hospitals providing as-needed care. Today, healthcare as an industry has no precedent: doctors are becoming employees of hospitals and clinics, and hospitals are being acquired to form chains. The leading pharmacy chains are on an acquisitions spree, some even entering into partnerships with payers.

Yes, healthcare has blossomed into many new and uncharted configurations. What has not changed is—healthcare is the most interpersonal of businesses. Everything we do creates or deepens a touchpoint between patients and caregivers. We are directly and intimately responsible for people's lives and well-being. We can derive a great deal of pleasure and professional satisfaction when we heal or cure a patient. However, the opposite is true when the patient is not healed or dies regardless of all our ministrations.

At no time in our lives have we felt so much painful loss of life as during the 2020 pandemic.

Each of us is part of healthcare's problems, and each of us can be part of the search for solutions. Our mission must be to assure that nothing like COVID-19 occurs again on this scale. It is a big job but I am convinced we can prevail, heal, and grow stronger if we collectively put our minds to it. As author-philosopher Philip Gabbard writes in his book *Thrivation*:

> And in truth, believe it or not, the fact that we exist here and now, today, is simply a fantastic testament to humankind's kindness, and thoughtfulness and mindfulness, and perhaps, just perhaps, if we could continue to work

together and continue to figure things out in a way that could very well improve the experience for all, and not just some, then we could actually, no ... most definitely, elongate the opportunity for our people, our kind, our species to have a piece of what we have today, but just a tad bit better.

I believe it will require you to be brutally honest with yourself and your colleagues about what has happened and what steps each of us can take to effect a turnaround. As we go to work on the solutions, I also believe we need to be very realistic about exactly what we can achieve and how long it will take to see results. We must be cognizant that there are many things we can change; that there will be some we cannot change or fix; and, in the final analysis, that we know which are which so we do not waste our efforts.

Bedside Consult: What the Healthcare World Needs NOW

From one continent to another, we are on an unsustainable healthcare cost curve that threatens our ability to bounce back from the severe challenges, both economic and pandemic, we now face. RHIT unlocks the door to the transformation of healthcare. We—the informaticists, clinicians, management engineers, senior IT executives, IT specialists, and the diverse talents of so many others—hold that key. It is we who must create the applications, processes, and workflows that improve quality, safety, access, outcomes, and which result in greater cost efficiency.

I am confident we can make this transformation happen. Why? Because many other revolutions involving technology in the workplace have happened over the past century. According to the Merriam-Webster Dictionary, it was in 1969 that the term "inbox" first entered the American lexicon, to describe a physical tray holding incoming paper-based mail and work documents. Over the next forty-plus years, the inbox has morphed into a technology-based tray where important messages and information are received, sent, and stored on our personal computers, handheld devices, and mobile smartphones.

The inbox is front and center in the story of how the world's manufacturing-based industrial economy was transformed into an information- and knowledge-based service economy, *driven by data and analytics.* The inbox tells the story of how savvy businesses began to share information quickly and inexpensively. These tech-savvy businesses effectively leveraged this information to deliver higher quality products at lower costs to a global marketplace. By meeting the needs of their customers while innovating to develop new market shares, these businesses saw their profits grow while their competitors' profits shrank. Smart companies thrived in this new data-driven marketplace while others, either unable or unwilling to adapt, could no longer compete.

Does this sound at all familiar in our healthcare business?

While most industries became more efficient and streamlined as a result of high technologies, healthcare in many ways remained frozen in time. In many respects, healthcare still operates like the typical business of 1969: largely paper-based, it ignores electronic information tools that can facilitate evidence-based best practices, and it functions without employing data and analytics to qualify and quantify the care we provide.

These economic realities are quickly catching up in our business, in large part because of change. Not the change we ought to have been gradually implementing for years and years, but the sudden, undeniable change brought upon by the COVID-19 pandemic, which forced us to change, whether we wanted to or not.

Yet medical decisions are being made according to implicit criteria—hidden internal knowledge from experience and intuition—rather than explicit criteria, the external, up-to-date knowledge that can be checked, evaluated, and updated. Books written by one doctor after another cite proof of glaring, unacceptable variations in how healthcare is provided and shed light on disparities existing in Europe, Scandinavia, the U.S., Mexico, China—anywhere, everywhere. Who is paying attention? Apparently too few: many providers are not taking advantage of twenty-first-century technologies to access twenty-first-century information, choosing instead to provide care the same way it was done some forty or more years ago. Who can dispute this fact when the huge fax machines stand on counters in every healthcare office?

Simply put, we must change from a paper-based system in which most clinical decisions are made primarily by gut-level or recalled judgments. In its place, we need to implement a system based not on one's recall ability and shift to a data- and evidence-based system. We do not advocate replacing human knowledge and experience; rather, augmenting it with the many advanced technologies at our disposal.

We must create electronic systems so easy to use and reliable that they make physicians want to leave their paper medical records behind. We must create clinical decision support systems (CDSS) that make it routine for physicians to cross-check their internal knowledge with data and evidence. We must implement workflow solutions based upon sound methodologies that continuously improve the efficiency of healthcare. We must make physicians want, yes, demand the enormous power that RHIT brings to the practice of medicine.

Never has the need for a transformation of healthcare been more necessary. It is the means by which we can profoundly affect positive change in four key areas: quality and safety, access to care, superior outcomes, and lower costs of care. You, the reader, are the leader who can implement the solutions we need to drive this transformation. By embracing and implementing revolutionary healthcare IT solutions, you can transform the way the best healthcare possible is delivered to our patients. If you do not do it, it will not happen. You must step forward, and you must lead. It is no longer about what others have done or what others are thinking about doing. It is about right now, about what you and your organization are doing to transform your healthcare processes, workflows, priorities, methodologies. I suspect that some of you may see yourselves clearly within this context while others may not. Let me suggest to you today that no matter who you are and what your role is, you have an important if not critical role to play in achieving transformation.

You can fulfill your role by building a multidisciplinary skunk works team with the desire and expertise needed to solve your particular problems. You can change your information handling from paper to digital. You can fulfill your role by gathering and sharing data and evidence as you go along. And you can fulfill your role by having the courage to stay the course or to change your mind—whichever the situation calls for. Great science comes from gaining new knowledge and perspectives, accepting that old paradigms and practices often must be replaced by newer, better ones.

The Pandemic, Economics, and Politics

I believe it came as something of a surprise to all of us just how profoundly the pandemic affected everything about our life on planet Earth. I believe that is referred to as unanticipated consequences. Here are three snapshots intended to help you focus on the solutions we must come up with.

The pandemic. Is healthcare to blame for our being in a pandemic? Are you forthright and tough-minded enough to answer that? Yes, of course we must bear some of the blame. But as I have pointed out, and will continue to stress throughout this book, this is not a blame game. This is a do-it-ourselves, let's-fix-it game. Each of us, regardless of our occupation, must take up the battle sword. We all see things that need to be thought about, reconsidered, fixed. So our ability to help extends beyond just our daily work in medical care, but also to our deep insight into how things work in healthcare.

The economy. Talk about unanticipated consequences: few could have foreseen just how profoundly the pandemic affected the world economy. Yet, in hindsight, the business downturn and the unemployment upturn pointed out how the single most critical success practice for any economy is the health of its people. Granted, fear played a significant role in the downturn, as it always does with any force threatening our livelihood or our lives, but the economy can be, and has been, affected by other occurrences—war, financial depressions, crises in energy, travel, and education—that have not impacted it quite as monstrously as has COVID-19.

Politics. Many of the social factors intended to influence our knowledge and opinions fall under the aegis of politics, because in every case some individual or interest group hopes to gain something from the interaction. The desired gain of these influencers is either for power or money. Modern politics pervades nearly everything, mitigating simple honest actions or reactions and undermining any sense of facts or truths we might hold. Simply put, politics widens the chasm between haves and have-nots in every way imaginable.

Dependable, assured healthcare, a relatively stable economy, and forthright, understandable politics are the three major factors influencing our quality of life. Many would say these are insurmountable issues to alter, but change always begins as a grassroots desire in hearts and minds. The belief that we can change the world must be acknowledged, and the challenge accepted. Once it is, adaptation to higher and more meaningful changes follows. Each of us is needed to participate in the reinvention, the new normal, of our livelihood.

After the CAT Scan: A Kondratieff Wave Cycle Diagnosis

Surely our healthcare processes need that CAT scan I mentioned in this chapter's title. There are changes underway already, part and parcel of the recovery from COVID-19, but like weight loss, lasting change will take time. There will be short-term gains—what the Kondratieff wave cycle people refer to as Kitchin waves—perhaps three to five years in length. And there will be the longer Kondratieff wave cycles, lasting anywhere between forty and sixty years. In between will be interim ripples from the Kitchin waves that roil and roil into Kondratieff waves. The point is, it is time to get started.

What makes Kondratieff thinking so pertinent for healthcare is its basis in technological innovation. While it is difficult to pinpoint how, or why, or when an innovation might occur, we can look back and see that changes actually do occur in cycles, whether technological, such as computing devices, or like the seasons of the earth. Cycles may develop of their own accord, as did the rise of government. But they can also be driven by a need for something new or improved, even simplifying or improving a human endeavor. What people have been able to create lifts the imagination, and hope, continually higher.

In our current circumstances, think about what it might feel like to have been part of one of these Kondratieff innovation curves that had a profound effect on healthcare. That is possible, and it is my purpose in this chapter. I believe we can collectively channel our intellectual energy toward fixing the problems in healthcare and coming up with new and better solutions for the work we do.

For our purposes, there are two types of groups: skunk works meetings for tactical objectives and working group meetings for strategy. Nominally, skunk works meetings are for short-term objectives—fixing things. Working group meetings are for long-tail discussions—anticipatory things—which are often broken out into smaller groups. Both must be planned, designed, and executed with great attention to detail in order to be efficient and meet their objectives.

Meeting design and purpose. Meetings are nothing new to us, especially when they are routinely scheduled and have no particular purpose or agenda. Skunk works meeting objectives are more tactical in purpose and can achieve their goals in the short term, like Kitchin waves. Working group meetings are like the rolling Kondratieff waves, especially when they involve fundamental or strategic change, and may go on for many months or even years, guiding the ship across ocean after ocean.

What Is a Skunk Works?

The concept of a "skunk works" grew out of a need at Lockheed to develop a new jet fighter technology for the army air force during World War II. The term itself may be attributed to the military's penchant for giving various development projects ambiguous but clever-sounding names, such as "Enigma" for the famous German codebreaking machine. Cloaked in secrecy, Lockheed created a workspace inside an aircraft hangar where the team met, in secret, to work on the design. The aircraft would become known as the P-38 Lightning. More revolutionary, innovative aircraft for the military and intelligence communities followed for years.

The Lockheed skunk works successfully undertook projects that the company's conventional aircraft development process could not achieve, in particular within the time frames the government agencies demanded. They were populated with technologically adept people to assure that the outcomes, while being outrageously innovative, were also realistic. There was strong, guiding leadership, but every team member was considered a key partner whose knowledge and contribution was essential.

Skunk works teams were small, often only a quarter the normal size. Reporting procedures were trimmed to the barest minimum, assuring a tight, rigorous focus on objectives and results. The idea of a skunk works bled into Silicon Valley, where technological innovation was created in garages across the Santa Clara Valley.

The working group. A working group provides oversight and is usually appointed for an extended period of time to analyze many organizational factors and make recommendations for overarching organizational improvement. Its job is not to fix a specific problem, but rather to assess processes: what works, what does not, how to realign those processes. Given its intent, working groups are composed of carefully chosen individuals who have demonstrated their intelligence and commitment to improving the organization over time.

Meeting members are often from divergent work areas in the organization so as to bring varying perspectives to the issues. This, of course, includes IT and often the CMIO, others from the C-suite, and systems people. They deliver high-quality thought and participation. In some cases, or at some time, a working group may split up into small groups to study different facets of a given problem. An added benefit accrues when individuals are multi-disciplinarily cross-trained, which generates deeper, broader understanding. When they report their recommendations to the group facilitator, a meeting is called so all members can weigh in on their reports. Everything occurring in the working group stays in the working group; no single outside arbiter makes the final decision on a recommendation.

Being appointed to a working group is often considered a compliment or even an honor. Healthcare organizations often create large, bureaucratic committees, when in fact those decision-making tasks are often more apropos to a skunk-works tactical solution. Working groups would be the more appropriate venue for solving problems (most of which concern financial matters) that have an impact across many departments or the entire organization.

Information technology and meetings. You should give serious thought to becoming a member of either a skunk works or a working group. The contribution you make is only commensurate with the value you receive in return. If you have that interest, you should be recording contemporaneous notes about what you hear, see, and think about, all the time, every day, all day, and want to address in a meeting. Ideally, use your mobile device to create voice recordings, which can be subsequently transcribed into text and sent to your colleagues. When combined with HIT statistical and analytical tools and database technology, the notes you generate from meetings assume an entirely different, more significant dimension. Those notes might be considered data at that point, but once entered into any sophisticated computer app they become information, and when put to use by members of the committee they become knowledge for decision-making. The added dimensions brought to meeting work by information technology are what Ray Dalio in his seminal book *Principles: Life and Work* referred to as an "idea meritocracy."

Your job is to disrupt. Harvard Business School professor Clayton Christensen published a book in 1997 entitled *The Innovator's Dilemma*, in which he introduced the concept of disruptive technologies. He posited that big companies could fail because they did not implement new ideas and accompanying technologies. This is still true. Yet in time, it became quite acceptable for a knowledge worker to become the disrupter rather than a go-along-to-get-along employee. Disrupters are the kinds of people you want in both skunk works and working groups. They are the brainstormers, the people who ask, "what if . . . ?" In most instances, you will also find the disruptions coming from the HIT people, not because they are troublemakers, but rather because working with technology has trained them to think about using technology and innovation to solve problems. They welcome opportunities to work with change, cause disruption, and solve problems.

Concluding thoughts. So far, we have discussed the *what* of many concepts. In the chapters to come, we will discuss the nature of *how* to work with those concepts, in particular how revolutionary HIT comes into play. As we leave this chapter and Part I, consider these suggestions for your meeting participation:

- If you are the facilitator, start and end the meeting on time.

- If you are an attendee, arrive for the meeting on time.

- Keep your meeting short like a skunk works, twenty-five to fifty minutes in length, tightly focused with breaks to think, process, and work.

- Have your meeting planned down to minutes per topic, and do not permit digressions of any sort.

- Do not be afraid to speak your mind truthfully, honestly, fearlessly.

- Respect differences, probe ideas, instill trust.

- Keep in mind this is a collaborative effort where each voice is equal to all others.

- Take notes on paper, and leave your phone off or at your desk.

- Neither food nor drink should be served; it is a distraction.

- Did I mention meetings should always end on time? And with a decision or plan for moving forward that is clear, concise, achievable, and will be decided upon at the next meeting. No stragglers!

The RHIT Interview: David Shulkin, MD, Ninth U. S. Secretary of Veterans Affairs and Under Secretary of Veterans Affairs for Health, Highland Park, Illinois

1. What was the most significant event or factor that determined your pursuing a career in medicine and transformational change?

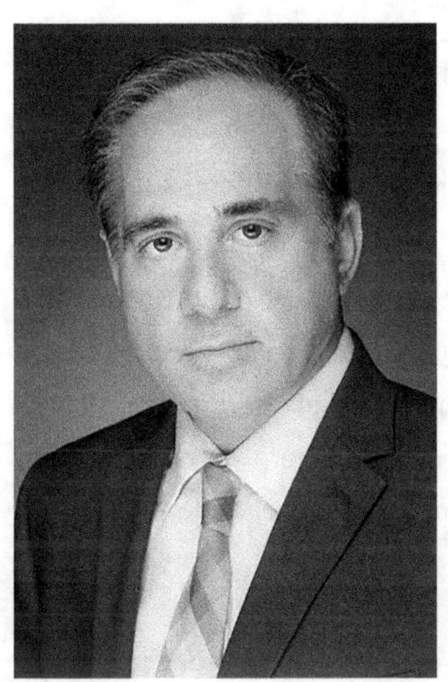

At the time I chose medicine, I was still too young to know what I wanted to do. I really wanted something where I could see results fast: a fireman (my real first choice), a policeman, a soldier, or a doctor. My mom preferred the latter choice, and so I made her happy. Once a doctor, I saw I could utilize more of my skills through changing systems. I was always attracted to creating solutions when I saw problems—and medicine was full of problems. That set me on a path to learn more about how our healthcare system worked, as well as how it didn't work so well. My early career was focused on quality and safety. There was much work to do, and much remains. If you can save one person and one family from having to suffer a needless medical error, then one's work is very fulfilling. The rest of my career has been finding solutions to our many problems.

2. After the pandemic is brought under control, what changes do you expect to see appearing in healthcare?

Pandemics change everything. Not that I am an expert in them, as this is my first. But we are seeing changes that will impact our society through changes in the economics, in the psychology of people, in our politics, in sociological aspects of how we relate to one another, and yes, most definitely in our healthcare system. We are seeing a greater need for people to be self-reliant, no longer able to trust their health to the so-called medical experts. This is going to drive more emerging forms of care, which are outside the mainstream of today's conventional practice. Care that occurs outside of our facility-based infrastructure. More healthcare decisions made by the individual, rather than the clinician.

3. What do you think are the most significant problems facing professionals working in healthcare?

Healthcare is still overly reliant upon human labor. Much like other industries have, healthcare will be—is being—impacted by technological efficiencies. Many of the jobs that are done today with many people will be replaced with more efficient ways to perform the service, with more reliable outcomes. This will change healthcare, much like it has most other industries.

4. What are the top three reasons you continue to work in healthcare, and how might that change in the next two, five, or ten years?

I find that nothing else gives me a sense of mission and passion like healthcare. Many people are fulfilled through economic performance, but for me it's about improving the performance of healthcare. I see a system of care that in two, five, ten years will increasingly allow everyone access to the best of what we have to offer. This will be done through improving access to knowledge through technology. I see the greatest opportunities in improving the ability to diagnose problems, then to match them with effective solutions. Too much of medicine today is really still guesswork. That's why we continue to see tremendous variations in approaches to common medical problems. We need to get better at diagnosis through genomics, analytics, and artificial intelligence. Then we need better precision therapies targeted at the cellular and genetic levels.

5. How would you suggest improving and reforming healthcare?

I used to think we needed to vote for the right politicians in order to get change. After spending time in Washington, I no longer think so. There are now many days when I really think we don't need to do anything to improve healthcare. It's going to happen, and it's going to happen soon. If we continue to operate healthcare the way we have, and only improve through incrementalism, our system of healthcare will be transformed by organized groups of disrupters. These will be people from outside healthcare who are tired of waiting for us to fix the inefficiencies, who cannot afford access to good care, who are tired of being denied access to their own clinical data. They are likely people who look at the world differently than those of us trained in the ways of healthcare, who know how to use technology in ways most clinicians do not. People who want to see change in the world. In my opinion, this is inevitable and it is good.

Part II

Transforming Today's Healthcare with Revolutionary HIT

"We are the change that we seek."

—Barack Obama

Change is hard. The ongoing pandemic has made it infinitely harder, and there is evidently no respite in sight. Administrators and clinicians alike worry about how they can continue providing high-quality care at an affordable cost to patients and deliver a suitable return to their hospital or practice, while at the same time absorbing the enormous amounts of new medical data needed to deliver that high-quality care. Doctors, nurses, and other caregivers know the healthcare system is ailing and must undergo a great deal of change to achieve the "new normal," but they have no idea how to do it without causing major disruptions to the existing delivery system. That is simply not an option.

Interestingly, many have professed to understand what's wrong with our healthcare and have proposed solutions. While it is always worthwhile to study and learn from these proposals and manifestos, more often than not they are very impractical to implement.

I have studied healthcare as a doctor, and I have studied it as a healthcare technology expert. My conclusions have led me to believe that healthcare is best changed from the inside, rather than with a massive overhaul. I determined that we needed what a computer-graphics designer refers to as an insertion point. It is where the cursor rests on the computer screen, awaiting the next keystroke or mouse click.

The insertion point as a metaphor for using computer technology was an inherently logical progression. HIT is mostly taken for granted by healthcare workers, but it is capable of so much more of an active role in reshaping the industry—one situation and one solution at a time, of course. That is our quiet but insistent revolution.

The four chapters that comprise Part II are intended to portray how to bring this much-needed revolution to fruition.

- Chapter 5 presents the first step, reviving HIT from its daily, often droll routines and challenging it to become a revolutionary force, working with us to bring about change.

- Chapter 6 discusses the process and outcomes model, with which the reader may be familiar, but integrated with our concept of change management.

- Chapter 7 proffers a new way of thinking about processes. There are too many interruptions and detours in healthcare processes; quality can become hit-or-miss and definitely difficult to measure or assess.

- Chapter 8 explains how we can use HIT tools and techniques to develop the transformational outcomes from our labors and get the clinical evidence and patient assessments essential to defining quality.

Chapter 5

Implementing Revolutionary HIT Change: The Chaiken Methodology

"In a chronically leaking boat, energy devoted to changing vessels is more productive than energy devoted to patching leaks."

—Warren Buffett

Clinicians, by virtue of their profession, want to protect patients: to do no harm. They always wish to avoid bad outcomes, especially when caused by new approaches or treatments. This tends to make them resist change. They will almost always tend toward using the diagnoses and treatments they know or with which they are already familiar.

Yet everyone knows that in any given situation there is likely a risk-reward synergy. What if two or three physicians—for example a cardiologist and a cardiac surgeon—argue over whether a procedure will result in success or cause greater harm? Which procedure has the chance of producing the most favorable outcome? Only one will operate; will the surgeon decide? Can they agree? If not, would the surgeon accede to another opinion? What if it is a crap shoot? Clinicians hate that.

In the *House* episode "Nobody's Fault," the brilliant eponymous doctor is the subject of a disciplinary hearing conducted by Dr. Walter Cofield to determine if he is responsible for best-friend doctor Robert Chase's being stabbed with a scalpel and nearly murdered by an out-of-control patient.

"My process is proven. Good things usually happen, bad things sometimes happen," says Dr. Gregory House.

"And when bad things happen, we should figure out what went wrong so we can learn from it, correct?" asks Cofield.

House replies, "So we can assign blame, instead of recognizing that bad things sometimes happen? It's nobody's fault."

In this very Machiavellian encounter, House is, as usual, iconoclastic, a revolutionary. He is portrayed as a clinician who is unafraid of taking risks or issuing shoot-from-the-hip outrageous diagnoses. He often makes decisions regardless of what other doctors think, or without consulting his team or any established medical references—either books or the computer—solely based on his knowledge and perceptions. House's more honest viewpoint is to accept that an error occurred and move on.

Cofield, the inquisitor, represents the righteous establishmentarian perspective, intent on determining right or wrong and who is at fault.

Chase does not feel it is anyone's fault.

The viewers, like House's resident staff, are left with three interpretations—we made a mistake, just forget it; we need to find out who is at fault; or it was nobody's fault—from which to decide which is the best outcome. But what makes for good television entertainment does not necessarily make for good healthcare. The reason for relating this rather lengthy critique is to point up the need for an open-minded, factually driven champion to lead the way to revolutionary HIT. Is this a role for you? Someone must be your fearless leader. If not you, then who?

Whomever you choose, your skunk works will need lieutenants to implement the change. The task cannot be accomplished single-handedly. You will need to enlist others who, like you, will regard this transformational change as essential and achievable. Each of you must keep an open mind, suppress judgment, and seek honesty and truth in what you are doing, because it is at the heart of our mission. Yet to achieve these very human attributes, it makes the most sense for us to found our purposes on scientific fact. That must always be the basis for our analysis and diagnostics, and is the springboard for our recommendations and game plan for revolutionary change. A demonstrable scientific basis is also the most compelling motive for convincing others to participate because we are, all of us, scientists.

I believe that a revolution in changing healthcare absolutely must involve HIT personnel. They, too, are scientists as well as IT professionals and are, by virtue of their nature and their occupation, agents of change. They can provide the proof of concept. HIT also has the tools and skills to establish the scientific bases for the changes we believe we need in our healthcare organization. This work has many facets—changing personal opinions and attitudes, devising new processes, overcoming institutional, political, and regulatory hurdles—and scientifically proving the change is the fulcrum. It will take time and much effort, but it will be worth it.

Evolutionary versus Revolutionary Change

Evolutionary change is what happens to each of us, all the time. Evolutionary change is gradual, often subtle, but essential to our growth as individuals, institutions—in all human endeavors. Revolutionary change is rarer, sometimes unexpected, often the result of an untoward event in gradual change. We are more cognizant of revolutionary change when it occurs, perhaps as something needed, but also because it is often an eruption that messes things up.

The revolutionary change for HIT I am proposing is nearer evolutionary than one like the French Revolution. In many ways, it is organic change, the result of many culminating evolutionary events such as a cure for cancer. A *revolutionary* change precludes the course of events returning to the previous status quo. Yet revolutionary change can and should be managed in sophisticated ways that evolutionary change cannot. Revolutionary change is the volcano erupting. Evolutionary change is the lava flowing down the mountainsides.

Here are a few simple illustrations of evolutionary vs. revolutionary change in IT:

Evolutionary IT	Revolutionary IT
Programming languages (e.g. COBOL, Python)	Modular app development
Device storage (floppy disk, hard disk, DVD)	Cloud Storage
Stand-alone computing devices	Blade servers, cloud computing
Data processing	Machine learning/ artificial intelligence
Client/server (mainframe to PC)	Mobile using internet

For example, programming languages evolved from COBOL and Fortran to Java and Python, and continue still, while fourth-generation modules were revolutionary leaps in programming productivity. Machine learning and AI moved the diagnostic from the doctor's data to the inference engine. Telemedicine was not truly practicable before internet access.

There is no question that medical research has similarly evolved, steadily and progressively: organ transplants, stem cells, gene therapy. Yet the immense challenges of the future we must address are not so flashy: increasing costs of care, loss of clinicians, increase in senior citizen care, and so on will require a different change perspective for the healthcare industry. My thesis for this book is, as stated before:

> *Revolutionary Healthcare Information Technology* (RHIT) offers clinicians, researchers, and administrators immensely powerful tools to drive clinical and administrative processes to deliver high-quality, safe, accessible, and investment-responsible medical outcomes.

A key to understanding the difference between evolutionary and revolutionary HIT is in the term *transformation*. Revolutionary transformations are soundly conceived and implemented with great effect. They are good to go. They are the desired outcome of both types of change. Change is the process and it is also the outcome. If there is an old, outdated applecart in the computer facility, our objective is to work collaboratively with HIT to upset it.

The Chaiken RHIT Methodology

A methodology can often provide the structure for how to think about initiating change and working through its implementation. My methodology was developed to express the functionality of the four tenets of the Hippocratic Code by demonstrating a new way to think about process and workflow. This is critical to its implementation.

Patient care is a function of each of a number of *processes* required to obtain an acceptable outcome. *Workflows* are made up of individual tasks undertaken by clinicians and non-clinicians. Each process in patient care is one of the processes of the clinician or non-clinician workflows. So patient outcomes, and outcomes in general, are the sum of all of the *processes* occurring prior to that outcome. It is also the sum of all the individual processes of the workflows that touch the patient. If patient care is viewed as a horizontal line, and the workflows are represented by crisscrossing lines that cross them, then each touchpoint represents a process that impacts the patient. This diagram expresses how revolutionary workflows crisscross processes efficiently, simply, and more economically for both the patient and the provider.

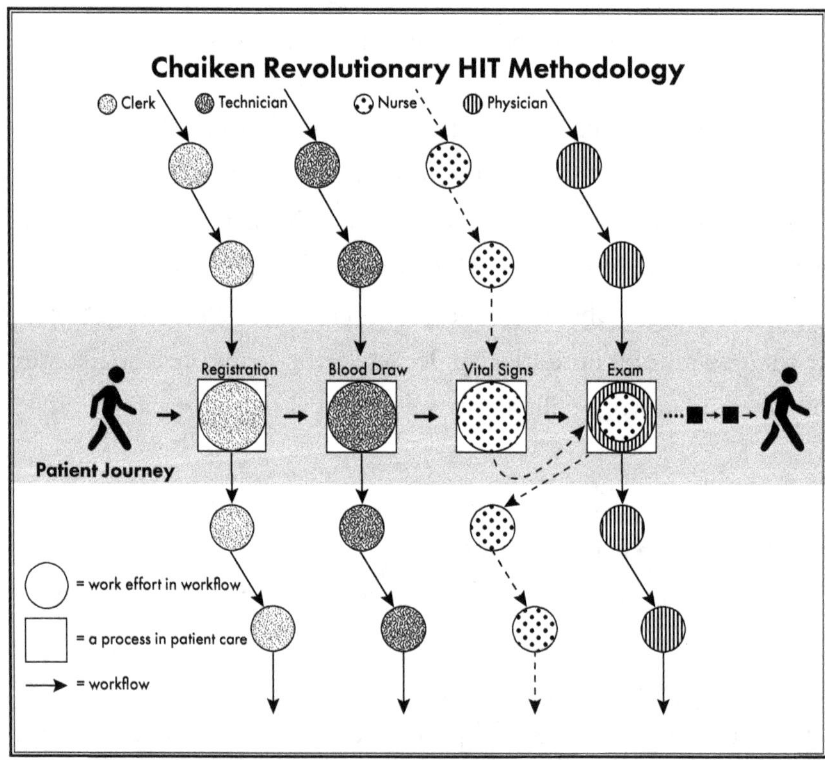

These touchpoints represent a medical or administrative procedure—an examination, a lab test, biopsy, completing an insurance form—an intersection of the workflow where the patient, a clinician, and often a staff member may all be involved in the process of healthcare. These touchpoints also represent Bruce Springsteen's expression of the *human touch*, which is the most important and is made tangibly more effective through the use of revolutionary technology.

Bedside Consult: The Chaiken Methodology as a Mathematical Expression

For the mathematically inclined reader, here is the methodology in formula:

$$\text{Work in Process}_m = \sum(\text{Work of Person}_1 + \text{Work of Person}_2 + \text{Work of Person}_3 \ldots \text{Work of Person}_n)_m$$

(Where work of one person expends her effort in her workflow to complete her share of the process. E.g., intubating a patient, whether the process requires one or several people)

$$\text{Workflow}_m = (\text{Work in Process}_1, \text{Work in Process}_2, \text{Work in Process}_3, \ldots \text{Work in Process}n)_m$$

(Where work in process reflects the effort of each worker in completing his share of the process. E.g., pharmacist preparing medications for patients.)

Total Work Effort = $\sum$(Work in Process$_1$, Work in Process$_2$, Work in Process$_3$, . . . Work in Process$_n$)

(Where the work in each process contributes to the overall outcome for the patient and where revisions and reviews—iterations — refinements can lead to a superior outcome. E.g., repair of an inguinal hernia.)

Patient Journey = (Process$_1$, Process$_2$, Process$_3$, . . . Process$_n$)

(Where each process is a discrete activity, performed by an experienced worker(s), involving the use of distinct specialized tools and skills, contributing essential quality to improving the overall team effort and, ultimately, the outcome. E.g., patient's diagnosis and treatment for diabetes.)

Patient Experience = Perception of Patient Journey + Outcomes of Patient Journey

(Where each process is a discrete activity delivering an administrative and clinical outcome. E.g., patient's perceptions of her care.)

Transformation

Everything—and I do mean everything—about achieving these goals is changing, rapidly and profoundly. I am sure you see it every day in your work. But most of these changes cannot be satisfactorily managed and rendered as transformative using today's stagnant, erratically performing business model. Fee-based services, "smokestack" treatments, outdated twentieth-century accounting, semitransparent patient satisfaction tracking, and the lack of an overall systemic strategy—all need to be scrutinized, assessed, and held to a standard of performance and delivery.

While performing "surgery" on these individual diseases, one at a time, may have appeal, it is not transformative. We need to transform the way we think about healthcare and use new (at least to healthcare) methodologies to transform our industry. If certain proof of why healthcare must take a transformative look at itself is needed, one need only look back at the 2020 coronavirus pandemic, wherein current procedures across the board either failed, fell short, or crashed with disastrous results. As Stanford economist Paul Romer once remarked, "A crisis is a terrible thing to waste." Of course, this does not account for the rampant change every individual on the planet is going through, every day of life. A crisis can present an opportunity to institute systemic change because its inherent stress makes the search for answers more of a priority. Choose your point of attack wisely.

Think of healthcare as if it were a garden hose with many kinks. Its processes form the workflow, a consistent flow of water. The kink is a poorly defined and ill-executed process that generates an undesirable outcome. A process is a step along the way in many individual workflows and patient journeys. A kink, or problem with the process, is when something interferes with the workflow or patient journey. Analyzing workflows and processes using HIT tools points out which processes are problematic and why. This has a significant impact on outcomes, but provides a way they can be adjusted, reassigned, or deleted. For example, if an individual nurse can perform a clinical process, why not reassign it from the doctor or the team?

Without analyzing workflow and processes, "bad" outcomes appear as symptoms and are difficult to identify, document, and address for improvement. In transformation, both workflow and process are strategically changed so that the outcome is holistically improved. Just observing the kinks in the hose is not going to work. Our objective is to straighten them out so the water flows in order to achieve higher-quality care, safety, access, outcomes, and smaller investments.

The most efficient un-kinking is to turn on the water and let it flow through the hose—submitting it to HIT's system analysis—fixing the kinks as it does so. And so can we transform healthcare from ill-conceived workflows and processes to better patient journeys. Clinical and administrative operations must be integrated into a workflow, with each participating in the overall process of patient healing and care. The criteria for this new workflow must be the consistent attention to the three essential outcomes. Revolutionary HIT is both the toolset and the technician-partner we need to get this done.

HIT has the diagnostic tools and experience to launch studies of broken systems and their purported workflow processes. The HIT people understand workflow, process, system analysis, and scientifically assessing outcomes. Many even have a sense of how HIT can, *should*, and, in some cases, does support business methodology. They have the technology and they are experts in its uses. It is unlikely a thoroughgoing transformation is possible without their full involvement. All they lack is the go-ahead from you.

Becoming a Change Manager

Every organization has differing policies, procedures, and politics, so if you are intent upon effecting change and transformation, employ your own knowledge, insights, and decision-making for how to get your effort going. The most important aspect is to avoid calling attention to yourself and your intent at first. You want as much freedom as possible, without oversight. If you must gain approval from your management, make sure you have a tentative written statement of purpose to explain your purpose. It need not be long, but ought to touch on these points (this could be presented as a simple memo instead of a bullet list):

- The problem: an absence of, or a dysfunctional, holistic system for, achieving desired outcomes

- What's working, what is not, and why

- What similar institutions are having the same problem and what they are doing about it

- How solving the problem can improve processes and work-flows while enhancing the patient experience

- How HIT can analyze workflow with HIT systems analysis tools and help, or design and implement, a new or upgraded one

- How improved workflow will benefit the institution (time, money, human resources)

- The solution: how you and your skunk works team intend going about the task and how long it will take

- Human and technical resources required

- Cost/benefit projections

- First steps: analyze the EHR's inputs and outputs

Here is a shortlist of prescriptive tips and information you may find useful in submitting your proposal to management:

- A walkthrough of existing workflows, making observations, and collecting data on the workflows and outcomes

- Gathering comparative information and facts from other similar institutions or software vendors

- Recruiting a small group (six or eight) of people for your skunk works

- Current state of HIT across similar institutions (meant to demonstrate competencies)

- Meeting with key HIT people to get a sense of possibilities and procedures; systems analysis of new workflow and tools needed to implement it

- Compare your institution's and HIT's org charts—do they closely overlay each other? They should.

Getting Started

EHRs are the first documentation touchpoint in patient workflow, and therefore an ideal starting point for our revolutionary change process. Through research and interviews with key players, accurately document how EHRs originated, are used, updated, and managed at your organization, and how one collects data throughout the patient experience. It is possible you will learn that both paper and electronic records are in use in differing workflows or departments.

In order to understand what change is possible or necessary, you need to take a look at the current state of recordkeeping in your healthcare organization. As you prepare your request, consider:

- The project may require a C-suite signoff. Ask your manager (unless you are that manager) how best to handle that approval. If they are reluctant to undertake that level of change, you might suggest a proof of concept project—for example, using the data captured in the EHR for evaluating imaging wait times in the emergency department.

- You may need to set up a preliminary focus group to obtain different perspectives and also early approval and buy-in. If you do, ask respondents to suggest their ideal means of solving the problem.

- The skunk works should include select individuals from disparate departments—for example, ED, cardiology, oncology, ICU, neurology, obstetrics, etc.

- Your skunk works' first project is to draft a brief survey and distribute it to everyone whose opinions are valued. Keep it short and simple.

- Collate the data and present it to the skunk works. Once conclusions have been drawn, submit it to the C-suite for green-lighting changes.

- With a sense of possible outcomes, launch a second survey to learn how other affiliated emergency departments are using their EHR data to assess those imaging wait times.

Once you have your EHR skunk works project operational, create a master implementation schedule. Senior management meetings are useful for communicating the new plan. Suggest to them that analyzing EHR data is only the first wave of implementing a revolutionary HIT system, which we will continue discussing in future chapters.

The RHIT Interview: John Glaser, PhD, Healthcare Information Technology Executive, Harvard Medical School, Boston, Massachusetts

1. What was the most significant event or factor that determined your pursuing a career in healthcare information technology?

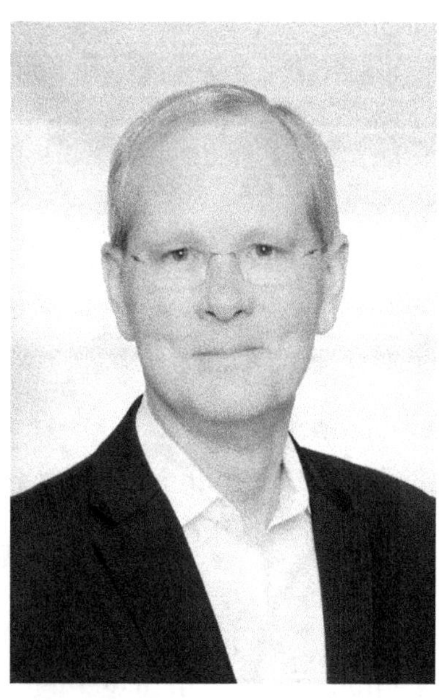

After college I wound up on my big life adventure hitchhiking from Fairbanks, Alaska, to the Panama Canal. I got down to the canal, tired of hitchhiking, and knew I was madly in love with this woman I had met at Duke. So I headed back to Durham, North Carolina, to be with her. I didn't know what I wanted to do. I thought, Oh my God, I'm going to wind up begging for coins outside a 7-Eleven.

When I got back, I took the first job I was offered, as a Fortran programmer working on a big study for the National Center for Health Services Research at the Research Triangle Institute. We studied healthcare quality and costs comprehensively; I was assigned to do analytics.

After a while I realized healthcare was really complicated and cool, but I didn't want to be a programmer for the rest of my life. My stepmother had been in healthcare informatics and suggested I get a degree in healthcare or medical informatics. So I stopped hitchhiking to be with this woman, whom I'm still with, and got a doctorate in healthcare informatics at the University of Minnesota. It was a little like Brownian motion; opportunities come your way and away you go.

2. That's an amazing story. After the pandemic is brought under control, what changes do you expect to see appearing in healthcare?

What will the new normal look like in two years? What's the IT agenda that goes with it? The punch line is the initiatives that organizations had before the pandemic will be the same after the pandemic; they will just be accelerated significantly. So, what might've taken ten years before the pandemic will now take two. Telehealth is an example. It may not stay at the same high level it is now, at maybe 20 or 30 percent of all outpatient visits, but it is still accelerated. And there'll be other areas, too. Value-based care will accelerate. Why? Providers will realize fee-for-service is highly volatile. Seeing the volume drop, they'll seek a terrain where the revenue is more predictable.

Value-based care provides steady per-member, per-month revenue. Providers will examine the appropriateness of various care venues. We will see more care at home and more telehealth, along with more remote patient monitoring. People will seek shelter under the wings of strong health systems that are more convenient, and may even be willing to pay for it. Providers have to be more thoughtful about creating value. Large healthcare systems will get larger. Financially distressed organizations will seek shelter. Managing costs is going to get more attention. Many states are constitutionally bound to balance their budgets—with declining revenue and increasing Medicaid rolls, they will reduce provider reimbursement further. I think there'll be greater cost-cutting pressures on the hospitals.

3. That's a lot. That's great. What do you think are the most significant problems facing professionals working in healthcare?

The stress level will remain high. As mentioned above, there will be an acceleration of change. And that's hard; there's more pressure on the professionals to take care of more people, at a time of greater and greater change. This acceleration is on top of the changes already underway in the industry—this relentless shift to value-based care.

4. What are the top three reasons you continue to work in healthcare? And in your case continue to write about it? How might it change in the next couple of years?

You know, I'm in it now and expect to continue for a couple of reasons. One, it's very real, it's very human, and there's something profound about it. I just think it is amazing and rewarding if you can help. It can be maddening but certainly rewarding.

The second: I do think about the real opportunity to leave the world a better place. All of us would like to be able to say, in our last thirty seconds, that "the world is better because I was here." Third, it's intellectually very interesting. So if you want to keep all the neurons firing, it's just pretty darned neat.

And last point, the fourth, is this: I get to work with some really extraordinary people, you know, colleagues like you.

5. How would you suggest improving and reforming healthcare?

If I could, I would accelerate it to get out of this fee-for-service and get us into value-based. I would certainly ensure coverage for everybody. And I would double down on efforts to help people adopt healthier behaviors and resolve social determinants that impede health. We will never solve poverty or homelessness completely. To have our level of poverty in this country, with so many people living on the streets, is just wrong. So, let's go fix that.

Chapter 6

Transforming Today's Healthcare with HIT: Systems Thinking

"Results are gained by exploiting opportunities, not by solving problems."

—Peter Drucker

Although he may not have realized it at the time, Peter Drucker's thought about exploiting opportunities instead of attempting to solve problems was, at root, systems thinking. When Drucker published *The Practice of Management* in 1954, it was a relatively new field of study. Management meant performing work in such a way as to make tasks more efficient and cost effective. The human element of work was not regarded as contributing to these goals; labor was a cost of doing business, in constant need of being reined in. The first experiments in studying—and manipulating—human productivity in the workplace were undertaken in the 1930s, and were thought to be akin to how raw manufacturing materials were handled. In one famous behavioral study, researchers learned that worker productivity could be improved merely by changing something—anything, even simply dimming or brightening the lights—but the intent was not to make work better (an opportunity) but only to speed up productivity (solve a problem).

Drucker was opposed to marginalizing workers. He felt employees were an asset to the company and should be treated as such. His philosophy included refraining from thinking of them as "blue collar" in favor of regarding them as knowledgeable, experienced, and essential to the business's success. His thoughts led to a closer examination of how business got accomplished, and to setting aside the term "white collar" and replacing it with "knowledge worker."

The Systems Approach

Humans do not seem to be innately efficient at organizing (which launched a new business opportunity for Marie Kondo). In 1960s-era business development, a more system-oriented approach to workflow and process was afoot. Commensurate with this new management orientation was the emergence of human resources and new, more empathetic attitudes toward employees. This emerging systems approach was nothing less than a new application for the scientific method.

Yet to Drucker's mind, what made a lot more sense was a strategy that turned a perceived opportunity into yet another successful new strategy or competitive advantage, rather than diverting time and energy to trying to solve a specific problem. Like our garden hose analogy, our process objective is making more efficient use of time, employees, and resources.

The task of carrying this organizing concept forward would fall to Jay W. Forrester, a professor at the Massachusetts Institute of Technology, and his theory of system dynamics. Forrester developed it as a methodology and a technique for mathematical modeling so that managers might better understand their company's industrial processes. (No kinks in the hose, so to speak.) Over time, system dynamics was implemented in policy analysis and other areas, but its impact on modeling information processes is at the heart of our need to understand it.

Bedside Consult: Systems Analysis and Design

First there were computers, and soon after programming languages. When an individual or a department needed to work with some specific data, a programmer would write a routine or program to satisfy the specific need or solve the problem. There was not a sense of workflow yet. And satisfying a need was how the electronic spreadsheet came into being. Dan Bricklin, a Harvard Business School student, found it tedious to handwrite (and erase, and rewrite) numerical data on paper ledger sheets. He enlisted the help of his friend Bob Frankston to create VisiCalc, the first electronic spreadsheet. It is a classic example of how Bricklin, the businessman, looked at a problem as an opportunity and Frankston, the programmer, coded one of the business world's most valuable software tools, which launched the computer-based version of "what-if" analysis.

Yet writing a program for a single task was pretty much like removing a kink from our aforementioned hose. As we in healthcare understand it, informatics is concerned with unrestricted, unimpeded workflow, which presents a Druckerian opportunity instead of just fixing a single problem. As Dr. Peck said earlier in this book, life is, quite simply, problems. It is our job to fix them. But workflow helps us organize these disparate problems in our search for an integrated solution. That is the true definition of opportunity for our purposes. We want every change to make an improvement in our processes, which leads to better outcomes, not simply getting a kink out of the hose.

And so we come to the introduction of systems analysis and design, a broad term describing numerous methodologies for developing high quality information systems or, as we term them today, apps. Systems analysis and design requires an opportunity (aka a problem), information technology (computers and software), people (knowledge workers from both business and IT), and the data to be transformed into useful, structured information to support business decision-making and workflow enhancement. In short, systems analysis and design provides a methodology and a platform for improving business processes.

Systems analysis and design rose to prominence in the 1970s, gradually offsetting the dominance of the plan, organize, direct, and control (PODM) management mantra, for a very practical reason: businesspeople, realizing the immense (and mostly untapped) utility of the computer, were asking for ever more sophisticated information systems to achieve business objectives. Yet in trying to explain what they needed to the software programmers, something was getting lost in translation. The resulting information system or software application did not perform as expected, or perhaps even completely failed. The solution was getting the businesspeople and the programmers to sit down together to analyze the problem and in the ensuing process come up with some designs for the application that both parties thought would meet the stated objectives. The designs, which were rough versions of the information system, were called prototypes, which could be reviewed and tweaked as necessary. Two upshots of this collaboration were a new IT position, the systems analyst, and the flowchart, replete with its own templates.

Although tremendous strides have taken place over the past forty to fifty years, the issue of clear communication between businesspeople and IT professionals still exists today, and may always.

Yet both parties have made significant efforts to understand one another, especially IT in learning business processes. Accompanying that effort, the analysis, design, and programming tools have become much more sophisticated, easy to use, faster, and more practical for business application. Rapid application development (RAD) and several other advances in programming tools were an outgrowth of systems analysis; without its design element, there would be no information engineering.

Healthcare enterprise, already a high technology–enabled business, views HIT favorably as a partner in working on solutions. Yet HIT is rather like the human brain: we use some of it most the time, but not all of it as much as we might.

At this point you might ask, what does all this have to do with me and my work?

The answer is, quite a lot. We could harken back to Drucker's opening quotation: we should, each and all of us, be collaborationists, thinking about opportunities—not problems—to improve our workflow and the healthcare environment. Applying a systems way of thinking about how we can improve our healthcare workflow. One clinician/knowledge worker who did precisely this might serve as a model for all of us.

The Donabedian Model

In 1966, just as management and systems were growing prominent in business thinking, a doctor named Avedis Donabedian introduced a radically new concept in medical care delivery that was founded upon what we could call scientific thinking: structure, process, and outcomes. Dubbed the Donabedian Model, it framed the physician's work around the concept of quality. His paper was enthusiastically received, and a book entitled *An Introduction to Quality Assurance in Health Care* followed.

In his thought and writing, Donabedian expressed the parallelism between the components of a computer and healthcare: input, processing, outcomes. Yet his primary focus was ever concerned with quality of care. Simply put, Donabedian said quality of care occurs when it is a synergy between the doctor, the patient, the healthcare system and its standards for care, and whether the final determination of quality care is determined by clinical outcomes and patient experience. Again, we can see Donabedian's input, processing, and outcomes as the skeleton for his framing the concept of quality with structure, processing, and outcomes.

As he thought, studied, and wrote, Donabedian's model came to be defined as the seven pillars of quality:

- *Efficacy*: the ability of care, at its best, to improve health;

- *Effectiveness*: the degree to which attainable health improvements are realized;

- *Efficiency*: the ability to obtain the greatest health improvement at the lowest cost;

- *Optimality*: the most advantageous balancing of costs and benefits;

- *Acceptability*: conformity to patient preferences regarding accessibility, the patient-practitioner relation, the amenities, the effects of care, and the cost of care;

- *Legitimacy*: conformity to social preferences concerning all of the above; and

- *Equity*: fairness in the distribution of care and its effects on health.

Donabedian was a progressive physician who clearly gave much thought to his profession and the manner in which medical care was administered. It seems clear he was a staunch advocate of the Hippocratic Oath and committed to doing no harm to patients. He advocated that computer technology and information systems were essential to healthcare and wrote, "Systems awareness and systems design are important for health professionals, but are not enough. They are enabling mechanisms only."

But to this he added, "It is the ethical dimension of individuals that is essential to a system's success. Ultimately, the secret of quality is love."

Quality, then, is the end result of gathering information from Donabedian's three components: structure, or context; process, or actions; and outcomes, or the effects of all three in providing consequential medical care. It is quality that can be posited, measured, evaluated, changed. And most important, quality is your personal and professional goal for everything you do in healthcare. If you feel it is not, then it is your goal to achieve. The purpose of this discussion of systems is to give you tools that will aid you in your efforts on behalf of quality. It is about more than simply being forgetful or careless. It is about total attention to detail, because the outcome of what you do as a clinician is saving lives. You know this. You may not have realized there were these clearly defined tools to help you structure your work to achieve a high level of consistent quality.

Today, the Donabedian Model is still as relevant and useful as when it was introduced. That is likely true because it is founded on a solid understanding of systems as reliable scientific structures, tightly integrated with the prime directive of healing human beings.

The Scientific Method and Systems Analysis

It may be said that many clinicians in healthcare define quality for themselves, but the use of data and performance methods are changing this dynamic. Clinicians may be unfamiliar with the

Donabedian Method, but will readily understand the efficacy of his seven pillars: they are principles with which we can apply a methodology, one established by another or of their own design. Doctors and nurses are known to assume that their work is partially art, partially craft. Yet there are hardly any undertakings in life or work that cannot be improved upon by a systemic approach and implementation.

There is no essential difference between systems analysis and the scientific method, save for the purposes to which each is put. A comparison of systems analysis and design, the Donabedian Model, and the scientific method reveals that the three share a great deal of commonality.

Systems Analysis and Design	Donabedian Pillars	Scientific Method
Conceptualize	Efficacy	Propose
Plan	Effectiveness	Plan
Requirements analysis	Efficiency	Research
Design	Optimality	Hypothesis
Development	Acceptability	Experiement
Test and Integrate	Legitimacy	Repeat experiment (by others)
Install and depl;oy	Equity	Use and observe
Evaluate		Analyze collected data
Revise, replace		Build upon discovery

The scientific method ought to be an important instrument in our doctor's bag. Healthcare is nearly pure science. Information technology has continually purified healthcare science and will continue to do so, if given the opportunities. HIT can help us, the clinicians, but we can also help ourselves and help HIT in the bargain by using our critical thinking faculties to seek ways to improve our systems and our workflow. Otherwise, there is no change. To do so is to think of these three as principles or ground rules for deployment with a methodology, such as my own.

In far too many instances, clinicians are not given the tools, information, or feedback they need to do the work of quality. If they were, then most would respond analytically and change their behavior. Over the past twenty-five years, information technology has gone far in changes in clinician attitudes. The practice of medicine is much more consumer-focused. Both doctors and nurses today are patient-focused, yet they still need the tools to do better rather than getting beaten with a stick to increase productivity and writing more and more documentation that offers no benefit to their patients or their clinical understanding. The enemy is the bureaucracy and the established "old ways" things get done, both of which are set in concrete and resistant to change. Enlightened organizations—and there are several—understand that healthcare requires constant striving toward excellence rather than improving profitability. Excellence delivers profits, but profits will never deliver excellence.

Changing processes informs continuous ongoing improvement; it can, and does, change outcomes, and that is the subject of our next chapter.

The RHIT Interview: Paul Barach, MD, MPH, Clinical Professor at Wayne State University School of Medicine, Detroit, Michigan

1. What's the most significant event or factor that determined your pursuing a career in healthcare?

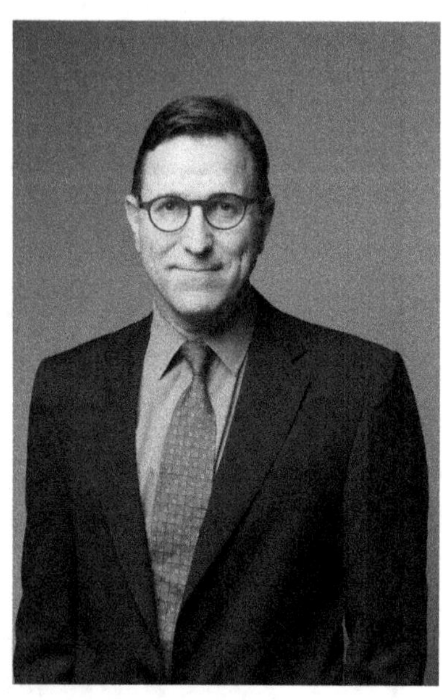

I think the most significant factor was the personal exposure to disease and sickness as a young boy. My father was a physician and worked at the World Health Organization in different parts of the world. That exposure early on fascinated me about biological organisms: when do things go wrong, solving the problems, reducing pain and suffering by people. I loved the intellectual pursuit of understanding why and how healthcare problems can be addressed, diagnosed, and ultimately resolved.

2. After the pandemic is brought under control, what changes do you expect to see in healthcare?

First and foremost, I believe we need to rethink the relationship between public health and society. Public health has taken an extraordinarily damaging blow during the COVID pandemic. COVID-19 has exposed the vulnerabilities of the nation's public health infrastructure and also revealed a failure to delineate the respective roles of the healthcare and public health systems, including shared responsibilities for emergency preparedness, planning, quality of care, and implementation. The narrative emerging is that public health got it wrong. Vital societies must have a strong public health platform. Without that, it's impossible to sustain life; from getting kids to school, having healthy babies, to maintaining modern commerce.

The second change is the increased value of health information—technology, telehealth, telemedicine, and everything around it—which is very exciting and remarkable. I think we need more realistic expectations about how technology supports and aligns with social values at a macro level, as well as at the organizational levels.

But technology cannot go rampant, so I think it's going to be challenged frequently. The organizations supporting technology need to solve real-world problems in the context of our values strategy. This problem is not a tech problem; it's a social-technical challenge. I think some really exciting stuff is going to happen.

A lot of healthcare providers were not treated very well. The inability of healthcare organizations to provide safe working conditions for their clinicians is inconsistent with the notion that safety is an overarching priority. Many will retire, resign, and leave medicine. The panic of politicians has put healthcare in a very awkward situation.

3. What do you think are the most significant problems facing professionals working in healthcare?

An incredible breach of social trust, growing anxiety, and burnout—what's been called moral injury. I think society is going to turn on healthcare providers as the pandemic evolves further. This has happened after previous earthquakes, pandemics, and disasters. Providers are accused of being too arrogant about their lessons, and are mistaken as part of the problem. There's a huge amount of internal dissonance: How could we be so vulnerable as healthcare providers? It's going to have a difficult impact on people who choose medicine and acute care professions to balance the risks against the benefits.

4. What are the top three reasons you continue to work in healthcare, and how might that change in the next two, five, or ten years?

I love the intellectual and moral challenges, number one. I love the ability to serve and take care of patients. I love being able to contribute to population health and how we help support people to fulfill their passions and dreams. I think that begins with a more ethical approach toward healthcare, and with better support for the quadruple aim: enhancing patient safety and experience, improving population health, and reducing costs while supporting healthcare providers' wellness.

It begins with having a different and honest conversation with consumers and patients through co-production and co-design; what I call radical data transparency. The 21st Century Cures Act allows patients and families complete access to their data. That's an important step in the right direction. It allows consumers to be more accountable, responsible, and actionable about their disease risks and health problems like smoking, obesity, bad diet, and lack of exercise.

I think healthcare executives are going to struggle because of misaligned values, corporate pressures, and perverse financial incentives. The emerging collective sense is that hospital executives are not supporting their staff's psychological safety. That's needed so that employees can speak up and deliver on their passion to serve. The hallmark of aligned healthcare organizations is consistently delivering measurable improvements in customer loyalty, customer satisfaction, and employee retention simultaneously.

5. How would you suggest improving and reforming healthcare?

From a service perspective, a science perspective, and a business perspective, it makes sense to listen to the customer and redesign the service around them. We don't do it with the hours of service availability, or through transparent use of data, or shared decision-making, or because of work pressures. We need to shift our focus on what is most impactful for the community and where we maximize wellness. We need to shift the financial incentives and hold clinicians and executives more accountable to these targets.

Science is about ethical, moral, and resilient healthcare systems. We hold people accountable to the quality metrics they care about. Healthcare executives are held responsible through ethical frameworks. The data and science are tools that support decision-making by healthcare executives. The question is, will the financial and political incentives align so that executives do the right thing? We really need to support these very passionate healthcare providers to enter a system that's ethical, transparent, and equitable.

There are different models around the world; I'm for a universal healthcare model. I like the Australian, Swiss, and Norwegian models. We know that in countries where healthcare is a right, citizens are more compliant, eat better, exercise more, and have more fulfilling work and contributions to society. They take more responsibility for their own health. I think healthcare, like security and safety, should be a universal right.

CHAPTER 7

A Revolutionary Process

"When I started to look at cathedrals, I wondered: Who built them, and why? The book is my answer to that question."

—Ken Follett, *The Pillars of the Earth*

Set in the twelfth century, Follett's novel concerns building a great cathedral, one that will not collapse as so many already had done in the past. Cathedrals, built of quarried stone, had a common floor plan in the shape of a cross, which gave parishioners a clear view of the stained-glass windows depicting significant religious scenes on each side of the nave. The cathedrals often fell to pieces, yet the stonemasons kept building and rebuilding the same way. As with so many problems, the solution was found in a combination of science and imagination: a redesign, the pointed arch (a V-shaped stone wedged in the center of the arch) and the flying buttress (a joint supporting the ceiling arch at the wall). As you can imagine, it took stonemasons generations, many iterations, and many collapsed cathedrals to figure it out.

Process and Revolutionary Process

Follett's stonemasons had no sense of a process. All they had to work with was determination and iterative trial and error. Today, we think through almost everything we do, individually and collectively in organizations, as a process to which we contribute our labor for the purpose of achieving an objective or goal. Think of process as an assembly line. For decades, a line worker did the same task, perhaps installing a part or tightening a bolt. Gradually, assembly lines changed and workers stayed with a car or truck for a series of related tasks. Today, humans work with adaptive robots to collaborate on assembling a vehicle, so the process has changed iteratively to produce better results. Earlier discrete tasking has changed to a rudimentary process, which with robotics became an adaptation and an extension of the earlier process. This is good change; it is evolutionary and an adaptive approach, but it is not a revolutionary approach.

To my mind, healthcare is nowhere near the level of process sophistication as many other twenty-first-century industries and enterprises. It is stuck with two archaic types of outdated or impractical processes. The first is trial and error, not unlike the stonemasons of a thousand years ago trying to figure out why churches collapsed. Trial-and-error process, often paving the way for new learners to grow in knowledge and wisdom, is closely allied to the scientific method because it begins with an assumption and takes logical steps to prove or disprove. All good scientists use this methodology because it works, up to a point.

The second type is everyday process. We do things this way because this is how we were trained. It is how we did them yesterday, and for a lot of yesterdays, and it seems to have worked. It is rote; it does not change because we do not think about changing it. His many shortcomings aside, it was this kind of thinking House hoped to deconstruct in his residents' minds. Today's healthcare relies too much on implicit criteria to make decisions about a condition, rather than examining the explicit clinical evidence that can inform decision-making. Using implicit criteria puts us at risk of using outdated or broken thinking about clinical work. As one physician pointed out:

> I go to the lab on Wednesday and come back so inspired. I've had these scientists telling me great things of new antibiotics, new antivirals, new *everything*, but we're making just incremental progress, you know? In five decades we've only improved survival estimates by five months.

Why old processes are obsolete. In many ways, it is due to the nature of our work: diagnosis and treatment are too often sporadic, unstructured, unpredictable. That variable in our process is unlikely to change: we cannot put all the diabetic or COVID-19 or heart patients on a conveyor belt for the same treatment. But neither can we continue thinking of their differences, such as genetics, age, or gender, as inevitable kinks in the garden hose.

Another mitigating factor in assessing process efficiency is our physical environment—the facilities in which we work. Our hospitals are modeled on Florence Nightingale's Civil War–era pavilion design. It resembles a hotel or a dormitory with its long halls, at first lined with rows of cots and today one identical, totally unidentifiable door after another. Over time, procedure suites and labs for just about everything sprang up like wildflowers in these big square boxlike buildings, hither and yon. The proliferation of these disparate points of care belied the emerging need for truly integrated, holistic patient care. Some hospitals, trying to create a more orderly process, put colored tape on floors to guide patients and staff from one diagnostic lab or procedure suite to another—or not. Getting a blood test, an X-ray, or an examination by a physician was akin to a grand, albeit random, tour of the hospital. The nurse or orderly might push the patient in a wheelchair from one test or examination or procedure to the next, from one hall to another, up and down the elevators, ad random infinitum, giving rise to one asking, "Why is the endoscopy lab so far away from radiology?"

The next generation of process and workflow. Think of process and workflow as first- and second-generation solutions in hospital design toward creating a more efficient clinical practice. They might be thought of as separate and distinct concepts, but they function best when they are integrated to work hand in hand. Process is talked about but often remains poorly conceptualized and implemented as an end-to-end set to deliver an outcome. Similarly, workflow is for all intents and purposes dysfunctional in today's healthcare. Everything done to the patient is treated as a discrete, unique stand-alone task. This may be the most difficult workflow kink in the hose. It is not conducive to modern, process-oriented healthcare. Making our way to a revolutionary process-workflow is our objective.

This book's intent is explaining how to implement a third-generation, revolutionary healthcare IT. We must get the kinks out, once and for all, and make more efficient use of a clinician's time and expertise. How do we do this? How do we resolve these difficult problems and overcome them with new, more logical yet more innovative treatment patterns? How do we restore a better and more integrated balance between clinical and administrative work? With revolutionary processes, designed and created with HIT as our partner, tightly integrated with a streamlined workflow. As I have said before:

Revolutionary Healthcare Information Technology (RHIT) offers clinicians, researchers, and administrators immensely powerful tools to drive clinical and administrative processes to deliver high-quality, safe, accessible, and investment-responsible medical outcomes.

In order to do that, we need to develop a revolutionary definition and expression of the scientific method founded on critical thinking. The best was to achieve this is with the help and involvement of your revolutionary HIT.

Bedside Consult: The Patient in the Chaiken RHIT Methodology

Satisfactory patient care is the objective of each of the *processes* required to obtain an acceptable outcome. *Workflows* are made up of individual tasks by clinicians and non-clinicians that deliver outcomes. Each process in patient care is one of the processes of the clinician or non-clinician workflows. So patient outcomes, and outcomes in general, are the sum of all of the *processes* occurring prior to that outcome.

The first step, the sum of the processes, as characterized mathematically (from Chapter 5), is stated thus:

$$\text{Work in Process}_m = \sum(\text{Work of Person}_1 + \text{Work of Person}_2 + \text{Work of Person}_3 \ldots \text{Work of Person}_n)_m$$

The first step is to analyze every process, to understand what steps make up that process. You use analytics and the metrics assigned to a particular process to evaluate, or to assess or to learn how that process is working. From that conclusion you can iterate and change that process as necessary. Perhaps this goes without saying, but this works most efficiently and effectively when the patient outcome is the sum of their particular processes. Bear in mind always that good processes deliver good outcomes; bad processes deliver bad outcomes. Good processes are best identified by the use of analytics—how all those processes interact with each other to deliver particular performance metrics or outcome analytics that can be used to examine all of the clinical or nonclinical workflows to obtain the most efficiency and recognize the most effective ones while disregarding those that are less than effective.

Remember, the processes provide intersection points with workflow, each a touchpoint. The process-workflow intersections may provide either direct patient care or simply perform a management function, such as printing a document or ordering a prescription. My methodology is built upon the complex nature of these intersections of the clinical and non-clinical workflows on the patients.

Typically, these are the human touchpoints:

- Reception (admin): confirming the patient appointment, insurance check-in, co-paying

- Nurse who collects vital signs—patient height, weight, blood pressure, prescription check, confirming reason for the appointment

- Physician directing interaction (in person or online) with the patient: conversing, collecting data, compiling information for medical assessment, documenting the patient medical record, advising and prescribing, and recommending a therapeutic or maintenance plan

- Physician concluding the visit with collegiality and human concern for the patient's welfare

- Debriefing by nurse to confirm additional action items

- Front desk checkout to complete any documentation and make subsequent appointments

Some outcomes are of a clinical nature—patient satisfaction, wait times for appointments, test results, and so forth, but they are far from unique to healthcare. That said, both clinical and nonclinical outcomes can be evaluated through analytics, with the expectation that processes should be considered as routine IT maintenance like any other software or systems. If they are not examined, if they are never critiqued by patients and clinicians alike to see if they work well or can be improved . . . you can finish the sentence yourself.

Critical systems thinking. How many times in a day at work do you think about or observe a process or procedure that could be improved upon? Likely this occurs several, if not many, times a day. Does it just flit through your mind, then you forget it until the next instance? If this is as far as you take it, there is little if any opportunity for change.

Or do you write it down, think about solutions for it, and submit it to your manager or CMIO for action? If you take each step, you are employing critical thinking. The downside is, this is a variation on the old suggestion box, and you do not know if anything will come of it.

If on the other hand you share your thoughts and notes with a skunk works—one either already in existence or one you and others establish—you are taking actionable, enabling steps toward revolutionary healthcare. Your critical thinking is now a collaboration with others. When HIT is a member of your skunk works, you have a partner in helping create actionable critical systems thinking.

Critical thinking is an established field of study in philosophy, with its roots in the dialogues of Plato. It is a college course and well regarded in science and business. Critical thinking is always based on logic and is not necessarily seeking out things that are faulty or wrong, but rather attempting to understand practices and processes that could be improved upon, using sharpened intellectual skills.

When using computer-based software and techniques, we use the term critical systems thinking (CST). The most common example, again, is the what-if analysis feature from Bricklin's electronic spreadsheet, which made it the first "killer app." But for more complex or difficult problems, other critical systems thinking tools are also found in project management, game theory, calculus, and mind-mapping.

However or whichever critical systems thinking tools (CSTs) you decide to implement, their use is not simply useful but essential to solving strategic process problems that need to be resolved. They exercise the brain in a structured way that lends significance to the random thoughts about things that could be improved upon, which inevitably crop up in our thoughts a dozen times a day. CSTs sharpen the focus and give us, free of charge, the ability to pay greater attention to detail, a prerequisite when deploying the scientific method. And they can help get the idea to iteration, particularly with the skunk works, much more quickly and efficiently. It is always the little details that make big things happen. Mathematicians think of this as chaos theory.

Strategic thoughtwork. Most of the strategic work—formulating the hypotheses and testing solutions—is CST, thoughtwork. Once the problem is clearly defined, it is time to invoke the scientific method. Then you and the skunk works can collaborate, right up to the fifth step when it is time to test the hypothesis. This is when you bring your revolutionary HIT person or persons on board. They can put wheels on the hypothesis with workflow and process design. Because HIT's solution development process mirrors the scientific method, you all can quickly determine how to solve the problem and test it. This thoughtful, revolutionary pursuit of a new way to solve problems and improve processes begins in your own thoughts and perceptions.

If you work with the Donabedian Model or something similar, you can give your skunk works project stronger legs by demonstrating its relevance to improving quality. Making this a RHIT Methodology project affords an opportunity for a test drive, lending purpose and structure to the project it might not have on its own. Structure also helps portray how the change wrought by the project can be integrated into hospital procedures and does much to validate the project.

For Donabedian, the critical success practice (CSP) focuses on quality, as should ours as well. Anything that weighs down our pursuit of quality weakens everything we do. Revolutionary process, workflow, and structure are based upon the RHIT Methodology and its delineation. The result is clinical knowledge, acquired in collaboration with HIT's systems solutions—which proves the value of our efforts and give us the ability to measure quality and demonstrate better outcomes. Most HIT deliverables, as are those from IT in other industries, are focused on quality. The auto industry has a term that exemplifies quality: fit and finish. What is ours?

The RHIT Interview: Ahmed Zakiuddin, MD; CEO, Digital Care; Project Director, RIHIS; King Saud University, Riyadh, Saudi Arabia

1. What was the most significant event or factor that determined your pursuing a career in healthcare?

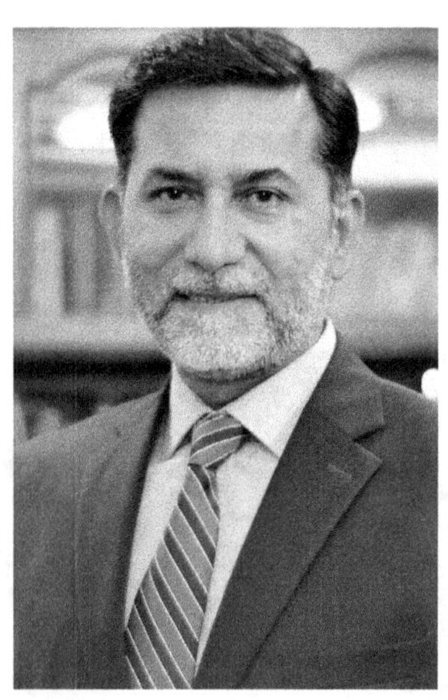

I wanted to become a physician at a very early age. The reason behind pursuing a career in healthcare was because I came from a family where everyone was an engineer. I think the major factor was the development and training of values by my parents; to live a meaningful and a benevolent life of service and contribution. I thought becoming a physician was the best way to do that.

2. After the pandemic is brought under control, what changes do you expect to see appearing in healthcare?

First, I think that healthcare will become a higher priority for the governments and NGOs. The global organizations like the WHO and others, as well as the public at large, are going through all of what we have.

The second is that the policy makers, regulators, and healthcare leadership focus more on the wellness of frontline healthcare workers. I worked in patient safety (in 2020), which is important, but so is the healthcare workers' safety. This is something which is very, very close to my heart. I've been working in telemedicine and digital health for more than two decades now. I think after COVID, additional health and virtual healthcare will become mainstream.

3. What do you think are the most significant problems facing professionals working in healthcare?

This is pervasive across different countries, whether a developing country like Pakistan or even the U.S. I think it's the lack of resources, human support, and material. Because of the lack of human resources—team members—and also the material resources, whoever is on the ground has to work more, which leads to burnout. Physician burnout is one of the top challenges right now in healthcare.

The second problem would be a lack of relevant training opportunities, especially for the soft and the human skills. I feel that healthcare professionals are not educated and trained appropriately enough to handle the stress of the job.

4. What are the top three reasons you continue to work in healthcare, and how might they change in the next two, five, or ten years?

Speaking for myself, healthcare actually provides me with the best opportunity to serve others and live a meaningful life. That remains the major reason I continue working in this space. The other would be the enhanced ability to influence other healthcare professionals and make a stronger impact in health systems due to my personal development as a health leader. After working in healthcare for around twenty-five years, the whole ecosystem has invested in me so much that there's all the more reason for me to continue working in healthcare. Now I can offer so much more than what I could have ten, fifteen, or twenty years back.

The third reason is something very positive and hopeful, the acceptance of a healthcare system for technology and patient centricity, both of which are very close to my heart. I'm very motivated and encouraged by that. Over the next ten years, healthcare challenges will continue to increase, due to the mistakes, the mess we have created, and the mistakes we have made in the past. We live with failed health systems and a very, very harmful lifestyle and dietary habits. The current model is not sustainable. If healthcare does not change for the better, the whole system will collapse. So, in the next two to ten years, I see challenges. These challenges are the dark of the night. But we are getting closer to the morning. That's my take on it.

5. How would you suggest improving and reforming healthcare?

You and I know what reforming healthcare requires. All the stakeholders must contribute and participate. So the first would be the policy makers, the government, and the regulators. They need to actually make healthcare more humane. Humanize healthcare.

I feel healthcare should be a hundred percent free and offered by the government as a basic right. But it must make economic sense as well. The policy makers need to decentralize and democratize healthcare. Community health and primary care should be developed, focused more on keeping in mind the double burden of disease and preventative medicine, which are both needed.

Healthcare should be the top priority of politicians and taken into consideration in all of their decisions and policies related to people. So, for example, regulating the cigarette or soft drinks industry. Any regulation related to those or to junk food, like McDonald's, infant formula, and carbon emissions. Every policy and regulation which affects people actually should be considered, keeping in mind the wellness and the healthcare priority. That's the first responsibility of the policy makers.

The second stakeholder is those in the professional community itself. They have a very huge responsibility for transforming healthcare. From a disease- or a physician-centric healthcare towards a patient-centric healthcare, giving rise to the empowered patient concept. If you do not put the patient at the center, healthcare will continue to be compromised.

So I feel that all healthcare professionals, especially physicians (who unfortunately believe they still control healthcare), will agree that undergraduates should be taught and trained in areas like leadership, ethics, emotional intelligence, and empathy, communication, collaboration, and teamwork, even sociology, and then definitely innovation and entrepreneurship. I think healthcare professionals must study these subjects, in addition to the clinical. Then we will make healthcare more humane.

And the third, obviously the people: the patient and their families. Each citizen should be made aware that he or she is the owner of his or her own wellness and is therefore the most important stakeholder. Every patient needs to be empowered. They need to take more responsibility. They need to be more informed. They need to be assertive whenever they're interacting with healthcare professionals and take part in the decision-making process. If we are going to transform or reform healthcare, these three stakeholders have to fulfill their responsibilities.

Chapter 8

Transformational Outcomes

"An individual is confronted by obstacles that cannot be overcome directly. In such a situation it is wise to pause in view of the danger and to retreat. However this is merely a preparation for overcoming the obstructions. One must join forces with friends of like mind and put himself under the leadership of a man equal to the situation: then one will succeed in removing the obstacles."

—The *I Ching*, Hexagram 39, "Chien: Obstruction"

There is good reason for the *I Ching* subtitle, "The Book of Changes." Two trigrams form the Chien hexagram. Each trigram represents an opposing force: symbolically interpreted, they are the abyss and the mountain, popularly interpreted as adversity and opportunity. The *I Ching* characterizes opportunity emerging from adversity as our vision being disrupted. We do not see the world as we did before. Think of order emerging from chaos. For most people today, the world we see is not as it was before. The adversity, pain, fear, and social disruption caused by COVID-19 gave us unexpected opportunities to seek out new ways of being, doing, living.

We have been challenged to change by these new opportunities, and that is good. As a result, we are learning to practice and manage healthcare in new, different, and better ways. These new opportunities are multiplying every day. Clinicians must, as the *I Ching* recommends, join forces—the skunk works—under the leadership of a change-maker, to recognize the "obstructions that appear in the course of time but that can and should be overcome." Are you this leader?

How Our Work Changed before We Knew What Had Happened

We clinicians work very conscientiously in practicing medicine to heal the sick and save lives amid myriad daily, ever-changing healthcare challenges. We produce electronic paper for an administrative bureaucracy that consumes over half of our workdays when we should be seeing our hundreds and hundreds of patients. It seemed like nothing was ever going to get better, while we were feeling like Doctor Langer, who said, "I just want to make [Lenox Hill Hospital] the best damn place in the world."

Then, in 2020, it got worse.

There was nothing inherently wrong or faulty with yesteryear's healthcare. It just was not as good as it could be, and had been like that for decades, if not longer. But nothing in particular was driving the mounting need to make things better on an institutional scale. Change was not the coin of our realm. We, like Dr. Langer, worked with, through, and around the kinks in our workflow hose to do our jobs. We were not satisfied with the amount of water flowing out of the hose, but it seemed we would have to go on accepting the kinks. Yet, in the back of our minds, we knew there was no aspect of our kink-filled workflow that could not benefit from closer scrutiny for improvement and, ultimately, some type of remediation. We must remove the kinks, eliminating the need for workarounds, which are the muscle memory of clinicians.

Then along came COVID-19, and leaving those kinks in was no longer an option. If we were to continue serving our patients, we had to change. A lot.

We have already changed, and are learning to be more adaptive to new conditions because we have to. COVID-19 left us with no choice. This is where we stand yet today, and although without a doubt we have come a long way since the pandemic first struck, there is so much more we can improve upon. For example, clinics and hospitals had closed, and doctors and nurses were leaving their professions, yet we who remained had to continue treating patients. We had no choice but to adapt, and turned to telemedicine. Like many other aspects of life, the internet and telemedicine came into play. Yet, in order for it to do so, a major kink had to be removed: not compensating doctors for telemedicine patient consults. This had long been a process kink in the workflow, but it took a pandemic to get it unkinked.

Telemedicine not only changed patient appointments—the input—but it changed nearly every aspect of the administration of healthcare. It is producing better outcomes, what I am calling *transformational outcomes*. To quote Dr. Langer again, to make Lenox Hill Hospital the best it could be meant believing "that IT is a huge component of that."

How we get from yesterday's everyday outcomes to transformational outcomes is the topic of this chapter, which coheres the previous three chapters of Part II and will prepare you to dive more deeply and enthusiastically into Part III.

Bedside Consult: Ancient Knowledge versus Intelligent Machines

The *I Ching*, now some 2,500 years old, is a repository of ancient knowledge used for purposes of divination. This knowledge is encapsulated in sixty-four hexagrams; each hexagram is composed of two trigrams, and each trigram contains three lines, which may be solid or broken. When both trigrams, or all six lines, are configured into a hexagram, it becomes possible to consult the *I Ching* and obtain a wise commentary, which, when interpreted, appears to answer the question posed to it. In the simplest interpretation, a question might concern a troublesome issue or a desire for clarity.

Yet the *I Ching* is also able to provide guidance about matters far more transcendent than a personal need or want, such as those concerning fate, will, a supernal presence, or a simple yes or no response. Given its basic configuration of solid and broken lines, the *I Ching* could be considered binary in nature—yin and yang—using the two opposing forces in much the way a computer uses binary code or on-off switches to perform its work.

Much the same is true of Go, China's greatest gift to humankind. Go is twice as old as the *I Ching*. Chess is generally regarded as a tactical battle between warring parties. Go is a full-scale war of strategy between two vast armies, differentiated only by the black and white colors of their round, stone board pieces. In chess, we attack the enemy to capture the king. Go is far more subtle. To consider the word *strategy* is akin to saying "thoughtful," "purposeful," "analytic." To consider the word *analytic* is to suggest the use of numbers in solving a problem. One analyzes, then thinks through the problem to a solution.

Which is precisely what a computer does, just a lot faster than a human can.

We seem to be obsessed with computers capable of finding solutions with analytical software. Early on it was plotting missile trajectories. Now it is artificial intelligence or machine learning. Why is this so? Because we are lazy; we offload any hard work we can onto a machine or device that will save us effort and time. But something tells us there are limits to how much we want computers to do in the realm of intelligent work—or even play. Some years ago, IBM taught Big Blue, its supercomputer, to play chess. In 1996, Garry Kasparov triumphed over Big Blue in four of six games. Today, computers have gotten smarter and routinely beat humans.

In 2016, a human and a machine played a game once again, but this time the game was Go, the most complex, strategic, and difficult of games. Lee Sodol, the human player, felt human intuition was more developed than Google's AlphaGo deep learning AI, against which he was pitted. In their second game, AlphaGo, on move number thirty-seven, made a move unknown to any Go player—ever. It turned out to be a brilliant move, which led to the defeat of Sodol, four games to one.

What was AlphaGo's competitive advantage? Its ability to capture and use vast amounts more data than the human intelligence against which it played. The same is true in healthcare: if our organizations are to prosper in our changing healthcare marketplace, we must acquire huge, objective data resources, analyze them, and strategically apply them to our processes in order to deliver the desired outcomes.

Data fuels analytics. Analytics drives process change. Process change leads to transformational outcomes.

All processes in a healthcare organization are related, as are the 361 black and white Go stones. Each stone is needed to win. While senior staff may monitor readmission rates and lost revenue, the readmission rate also relies on the effectiveness of many: the environmental services staff, surgeons, nurses, and others.

In Go, attention to detail is essential; losing track of one stone can result in the entire army being captured. Similarly, examining only a single healthcare factor fails to realize the potential gains that can accrue when there is a change in processes and workflows.

In Go, a winner is determined when one player has captured the opponent's territory, or eye, and has rendered him unable to make a strategic move. In healthcare organizations, only an enterprise-wide analytics approach can identify the essential improvement opportunities that enhance our competitive position in the healthcare market.

The Outcome

An outcome is the consequence of an act or multiple associated actions. The World Health Organization has stated that any change in the health of an individual or in groups of people that can be attributed to a medical intervention can be measured. Outcome measures—such as patient safety and experience, mortality, readmission, responsive and effective care—are all data-based and can be used in measuring outcomes, specifically quality of care, access to healthcare, and providing cost-effective medical care and services. These are outcomes our entire healthcare industry is working to improve.

Words are insufficient to express how deeply clinicians care about outcomes. They rejoice when a procedure is successful. They weep and mourn when a patient dies. There is no other profession in which lives are so in the balance of someone else's care. In a word, the term *outcome* is the expression of the quality and safety of care that preceded it. Yet there may be a disconnect between the clinician's sense of a successful outcome and outcomes that conform to misappropriated metrics.

COVID-19 strained healthcare at its every seam, and burst many of those seams. It lived up to its appellation: pandemic, a widespread (pan) epidemic (demic) of completely unmanageable proportions. Healthcare's response was as good or better than anyone might have hoped for, and that gave us pause to reflect on how much worse it could have been. It was indeed a major obstruction to our staid work practices, and by its nature drove us to major reconsiderations of our life on Earth. That said, some countries did a better job of containment than others. But long-tail, COVID-19 became the impetus behind the emergence of transformational healthcare outcomes.

Transformational Outcomes

There have been many quite thoughtful improvements proposed, intended to move from indeterminate outcomes to those that sustain honoring the Hippocratic Code and are based increasingly on good science. What is often lacking is a systemic workflow to support and integrate these solutions to providing better outcomes: transformational outcomes. As the word itself implies, a transformational outcome is truly what we in healthcare strive for in everything we do. It is not magic, nor is it random or accidental; it is built upon computer-based data, using the tools of revolutionary healthcare IT, administered by technologically skilled clinicians.

We do not need to tear up the entire practice of medicine to achieve transformational outcomes. We only need to refine and systematize what we do on a daily basis with a more focused intention on the transformational outcome. We assess our process, if we have one, with the intent of eliminating the kinks in its hose and improving the flow. We see each kink, not as an adversary, but as an opportunity to improve. But we need the help of our revolutionary HIT people and services to achieve this. There are two types of concern inhibiting transformational outcomes: clinical and administrative.

Clinical transformational outcomes. The transformational outcome occurs when the clinician is:

- Focused most on quality of care,

- Practicing evidence-based medicine,

- Providing documentation with the highest level of attention to detail, and

- Systematically employing state-of-the-art healthcare information technology.

Administrative transformational outcomes. Healthcare administration is constantly challenged by changing social needs and business practices that often put cost accounting before administering essential care. Among the many battles it must contend with are:

- Tightening business partnerships and governmental payouts

- Increasing operational costs

- Staffing

- Pay-per-service

- Privacy and records security

- Inconsistent patient outcomes

- Regulations

It might seem like all these different kinks in the hose are despairingly difficult to surmount. So it may surprise you to learn that they can be remediated collectively—not in one fell swoop, but as aspects of a new process, a new neurosystem. This is at the essence of transformational outcomes, which will guide healthcare to an optimal, new, all-inclusive transformational outcome. It will require change; it will not always be easy, but through a streamlined repurposing it will create a revolutionary healthcare enterprise. Telemedicine is an example.

2020: a revolution in telemedicine. The expanding implementation of telemedicine in 2020 is an example of a combined clinical and administrative transformational outcome. It integrated good medical practice with sound science and with IT's technological systems analysis and design. It also displayed a consistent workflow methodology that was essentially absent in the former office-appointment business model.

Telemedicine, at once more intimate and practical, has sustained and in many cases improved the quality of patient-doctor interaction; it has assured safety of care because the patient remained at home; access was vastly improved because web-based appointments were prompt and did not require travel or waiting; and the costs of an office visit were, for all intents and purposes, reduced or eliminated for both the patient and the organization without affecting doctors' fees. It streamlined the process, from creating an appointment all the way to delivering service to capturing patient outcomes.

Needless to say, the office-appointment business procedure had many obstructions, and we are innovatively streamlining and clearing many other bureaucratic obstructions that cost time, money, and churn every day. As the Chien hexagram in the *I Ching* states, "An obstruction . . . is useful for self-development. This is the value of adversity."

Transformational HIT for Better Outcomes

The most-used means of disseminating diagnoses, treatments, or outcomes is clinician to clinician, sometimes one-on-one, sometimes in department meetings, and in random conversations. These are not transformational; that requires an RHIT implementation. Data collection and utilization is assuredly central to this, because it is factual and can be dispassionately analyzed by the clinician using the scientific method. How, then, is the data accessed and utilized? Again, often only randomly: the clinician setting fingers to a computer keyboard, reviewing the patient data in a clinical chart, getting what she sought, and closing the screen. A transformational outcome would be driven by the embedded sharing of information in the workflow that achieves a change in clinical care. This information is delivered to the clinicians at the touchpoint where it is appropriate to influence the care. Why? Because a transformational outcome is the integration of medicine's scientific method in treatment with HIT's systems analysis, which facilitates *repeatable workflows and processes* throughout the medical facility.

Transformational outcomes reflect the highest expression of the art and science of medicine, supporting the businesslike management of healthcare. The outcome we seek is capturing data that can be reused. We call that a knowledge base. To achieve that, we need HIT's expertise and involvement.

The RHIT Interview: David Nash, MD, MBA, Founding Dean Emeritus at Jefferson College of Population Health, Philadelphia, Pennsylvania

1. What was the most significant event or factor that determined your pursuing a career in quality and population health?

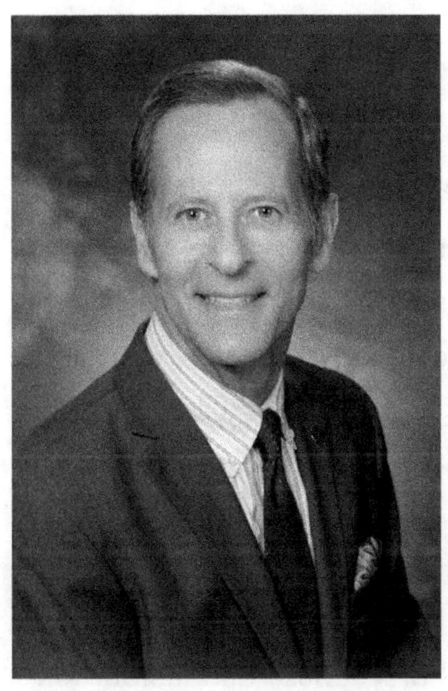

So, I would say three years of residency and a year at Wharton. We're talking forty years ago. I needed an explanation for why we were constantly readmitting the same people and making the same mistakes over and over. I couldn't understand this because I had no systems training. I had to go to business school to learn what a "system" was. Once I got systems training, the light went on. Right? Amazing. I thought, am I the only one who gets this? Once I understood the systems nature of care, which paradoxically wasn't taught in any aspect of medical school or training, I said: "Okay, there must be a way to fix this."

Around that time, Don Berwick came to campus. He was still a pediatrician at Harvard Pilgrim Healthcare. He gave a talk and I thought, okay, there's a future in doing this kind of stuff. I also met Brent James about the same time. We had a long ride in a limousine and Brent said to me, "This is what you should do." Okay, I thought. But it was business school that flipped the switch.

2. After the pandemic is brought under control, what changes do you expect to see appearing in healthcare?

Well, there's what I hope for and what I expect. So here's what I've been writing about; if people think this healthcare system of ours, tipping on the precipice of disaster, is going to take us into the future, then good luck. And I'm worried that is the plan.

But I'm hoping we'll have a totally different view and think about the business we're really in. You know, achieving and maintaining health. I don't think most people believe that. I think most are looking to increase market share by merging with hospitals, which are failing due to COVID. And I think they want to restart the utilization engine as fast as possible because of the incredible losses.

I would hope this is an opportunity to totally reorient what healthcare is here to do. Maybe technology can help with that. I hope that could be part of your book. I'm hopeful we'll take another look at building the bridge between health and healthcare because, as you know, Barry, our college was all about building that bridge.

We need to help people understand that healthcare and health are not the same. And in a city like Philadelphia with five medical schools, with poverty and crime and drug abuse and murder rates and all the rest, we must call attention to what people don't want to talk about. The pandemic has shined a light on this, which has been a huge help. Our enrollment is up. Much more attention is being paid to the issues we started legitimately talking about ten years ago.

3. What do you think are the most significant problems facing professionals working in healthcare?

Post-pandemic, I think we're underestimating the effect of post-traumatic stress disorder. The rise of PTSD in the healthcare workforce is a gigantic iceberg problem. I would make it the number one and number two problem. Look what happened without systems training; we had psychiatrists, house officers, and others thrown into adjusting ventilator settings.

In March and April, we were caught flat-footed—no crash training, no systems training, and no understanding of the greater place where they fit. It was a total catastrophe in New York and elsewhere.

So two things: number one is post-traumatic stress, and two is the need for a new Flexner report, which will totally reorient UME and GME. There are a handful of medical schools tackling this right now: Kaiser's Tyson Medical School and Geisinger Commonwealth School of Medicine (I'm a board member of GCS). So a handful of medical schools have figured this out, but until it's mandatory and on the boards, no one will pay attention.

4. What are the top three reasons you continue to work in healthcare, and how might that change in the next two, five, or ten years?

No, I'm not retiring yet. Top three: mental illness, mental illness, mental illness. I haven't changed my tune on this.

But the number one reason is being with students, training the leaders of tomorrow. I get my energy from young people; being around them keeps me going. This is my thirtieth anniversary on the faculty at Thomas Jefferson University.

Reason two is having the opportunity to utilize my network for good, to connect people. That's a huge amount of what I do. Three, I help a lot of companies that otherwise wouldn't really be connected.

I think about how to apply technology to all these problems. So being with students, training leaders, helping companies—it's a real privilege and a truly unique opportunity to be Emeritus, and have the autonomy to do these things.

5. How would you suggest improving and reforming healthcare?

How could any country invest three and a half trillion dollars and get walloped by a pandemic for which we should've been much better prepared? Every system is perfectly designed to achieve exactly the results it gets. Right? So tear up the playbook and start over. Nobody really wants to hear that, but in their hearts they know it's true.

Where should they start? Undergraduate medical education, day one. What's the system? What's epidemiology? What's an R naught? What are the social determinants and why are we here? That's pretty basic, instead of "Here's the Krebs cycle. You'd better learn it so you can repeat it tomorrow."

Part III

Applied Change Management

"The greatest danger in times of turbulence is not the turbulence; it is to act with yesterday's logic."
—Peter F. Drucker, *Managing in Turbulent Times*

By this point you should be well aware that this book is, at its core, about change, and more specifically the management of change. Unmanaged change is counterproductive. Managed change allows us to improve our system, get better at our work, and become more financially sound. In Chapter 3, I characterized two types of change:

Disruptive change is like working in the ED. You never know what the next patient's problem will be: a heart attack, a cycling accident, a blood clot, pneumonia.

Insistent change develops over time, like hypertension, a tumor, or arthritis. It is usually evident due to its increasing symptoms, which is why it is often ignored until it cannot be ignored any longer.

We in healthcare deal with both types, all the day long. Both can be managed if we choose to pay attention. For this reason

I introduced the concept of a changepoint, an uncommon and remarkable moment when your realization of some thing or event has changed, or is about to, or should. In such a moment, one would hope to recognize the change as an incongruity, a matter requiring attention, a serious problem. It has become something that needs to be dealt with, not swept under the proverbial rug. The changepoint recognition is the point at which you begin thinking about ways to mitigate the change. Ideally, you would formalize your thoughts in written form, then raise the issue with the team at the next skunk works meeting. That would be the beginning of a change process in your organization: recognition, considerations, solutions. In a word, managing the change.

Having read this far, you are likely ready to become engaged in roll-up-the-sleeves change management. The next four chapters describe, in my estimation, four fundamental operational issues in healthcare requiring applied change management. They explore and explain how healthcare professionals, whether clinical or administrative, can partner with revolutionary HIT to implement change management practices. But first . . .

What Do We Mean When We Talk about Applied Change Management?

Change is the coin of the realm in healthcare. Our work is erratic, unpredictable, unsettling, and all too often frustrating. We often feel swept up in a maelstrom of patient problems and their needs for our attention. Right now. We do our best, but it is day-to-day crazy time and it does not give us much time to reflect on how we could make our work go more smoothly. Does this mean we cannot manage change? No, it does not. But it does mean we must find and take the time to bring these issues in need of change to the attention of concerned others. First, we have to change the way we think about and focus our thoughts and energies toward positive change. That is the essence of change management, and it is simpler than you might expect.

Change management is a strategy. It is the means to your desired outcome. It begins with clear thinking and an accurate representation of the issue or problem that needs resolution. For most of us, that means writing it down, whether by hand or on a computer screen. This not only helps clarify your own thinking, but it is the best way to gain the interest and attention of others. To get yourself started, write:

- What was the changepoint?

- Describe the problem.

- How will change management address the problem?

- List possible applied solutions.

Now the matter has moved from a nagging emotion, such as "Why do we have to wait so long for COVID-19 testing results?" to a fact-finding project that can be worked at and logically managed until its solution is found. Change management methodologies have been devised by thoughtful people for solving problems; review several (or read reviews) to begin with, as reviewing and evaluating may help you more closely define your change management process. Some are available as off-the-shelf software; others come from consultancies, but one or more is ideal for you and your skunk works team. Of course, I hope you will consider mine. But whether you hire a consultancy, purchase a software solution, or design your own, the steps are similar:

- Plan every step and test the process.

- Organize your skunk works and support team.

- Manage your people; assign tasks and responsibilities.

- Measure: be prepared to demonstrate progress and results.

- Be a leader and appoint others; assure C-suite buy-in.

- Communicate, train, and support; repeat, repeat.

- Give your change management initiative a title and develop it as a continuous improvement methodology.

Change management is your skunk works. It is unrealistic to think you can implement a change management initiative by yourself. If you already have a skunk works in place, present your issue at a meeting and gain the group's perspectives and support. Once the skunk works determines its viability, ask for support from the CMIO, CNIO, or CIO, which is essential. Break the issue down into manageable steps with a timeline for achievements. Those who achieve the most are those who accumulate small, incremental successes.

The four chapters that make up Part III present change management (CM) strategies for four critical-path concerns, with a step-by-step guide to implementing a CM strategy. Think of these four chapters' highlighted bullets as transparency overlays, one atop another:

- Chapter 9 (the first transparency) describes how to recognize the changepoint as the first step in acknowledging the need to change outmoded, inefficient patterns. Changepoints initiate the opportunities for change management. This begins at the ground-floor remediation of processes into a more efficient, highly integrated workflow.

- Chapter 10 (the second transparency) presents reasons to implement change management so as to improve clinical workflow. A practical, structured workflow helps tame randomness and chaos and delivers a sense of well-being and job satisfaction to clinical workers.

- Chapter 11 (the third transparency) discusses how clinicians need to be informed and educated about change management implementation. They must understand that surpassing today's "good enough" is essential to superb patient outcomes and the continued viability of the enterprise.

- Chapter 12 (the fourth transparency) explains how healthcare lacks a clear understanding of how patients regard it, from the individual to the institution. Change management is the correction of misperceptions, creating patient engagement and building community: becoming an extension of family to the patient. Once medical services are redesigned as a workflow process, this becomes more achievable, a medical version of customer relationship management (CRM).

Chapter 9

Applied Change Management: From Stand-Alone Processes to Integrated Workflow

"Imagine that virtually everything important going on in your company can be captured as data, and that you can build algorithms to instruct the computer, as you would instruct a person, to analyze that data and use it in the way you agreed it should be used."

—Ray Dalio, *Principles*

Everything that can be managed is either managed or being considered for management. This is because humans want to be in control. Change management is a strategy for getting things under control. For healthcare, that means a reassessment of processes in favor of a more contemporary, profoundly integrated, process-oriented workflow. (A more in-depth discussion of workflow follows in Chapter 10.)

Thirty years ago IT told the business world, including healthcare, that their horizontally integrated business model was outdated. Business consultants such as Christensen and Porter had long before bemoaned healthcare's clumsy inefficiencies, but nothing significant ever changed. Service lines were, and are, established not so much for patient care as to generate revenue or increase budget. Their primary purpose was, and remains, to contribute to overall organizational growth. Unfortunately for the bean counters, the emphasis in healthcare has shifted dramatically to patient outcomes.

Bedside Consult: When in Crisis Mode, Follow the Data

March 2020. I am confronted with a world turned upside down. The COVID-19 pandemic has changed every part of my daily routine, limiting my trips to the grocery store, physically distancing me from family, friends, and colleagues, and forcing me to work from home. I have learned to adjust to my new work environment, substituting in-person meetings with video conferences, finding other sources of entertainment, and developing work strategies that make me feel less isolated.

I suspect this experience will fundamentally change how we all, the knowledge workers of the world, do our work and interact with each other. Yet this unprecedented event has also taught me a valuable lesson. While I always believed data to be a valuable tool to guide science and decision-making, I never realized how important a role it plays during a crisis.

During a healthcare crisis, the cost of being wrong increases exponentially. Poor decisions can lead to preventable suffering, unnecessary deaths, and wasted resources. Circumstances change rapidly, often outpacing the ability of managers to process new information. Relying on expertise built from years of experience becomes less valuable, as that expertise does not include consideration of the unknown and unanticipated outcomes.

When faced with a crisis, the importance of data literacy and embracing a data culture is critically important. Every decision, in addition to its heightened importance, also attracts additional scrutiny. Data analytics provides managers with a new set of information that helps them make more objective decisions. It further describes the current state and provides insights into the new reality.

Without data literacy, management may fail to understand the amount of useful information that can be extracted from data, and in turn may end up making decisions based more on intuition or guesswork and less on facts. In a crisis, "gut-instinct" decisions often lead to mistakes and unsatisfactory outcomes that are not easily reversed.

During a crisis, more desirable outcomes are driven by an enterprise-wide deployment of analytics, coupled with a workforce firmly grounded in data literacy and data culture. This allows organizations to leverage existing data sources such as EHRs, enterprise resource planning (ERP) software, and other transactional systems to extract and analyze the data. The information it produces can be shared with interested clinicians and leaders by employing dashboards.

The application of data literacy across a data-driven culture also offers significant benefits during normal times. Organizations can leverage their improved decision-making to impact clinical and financial outcomes, for example enhancing patient safety or decreasing treatment costs. Data analytics facilitates informed management—a powerful foil for both the common challenges facing provider organizations and unanticipated "black swan" events, such as our recent pandemic.

A vertically integrated business model was seen as more enabling and productive for business—and healthcare is as much a business as automakers or Amazon. A vertical, rather than the old-fashioned horizontal, integration enables managers to track every stage in the business process as well as build out with the same model. In 2020, Semantic Scholar Jessica J. Heeringa wrote in the *International Journal of Integrated Care* that "evidence suggests that organizational structures, composition, and other characteristics influence cost and quality performance."

From an IT perspective, vertical integration makes information transparent and available across different systems, regardless of organizational boundaries: clinical or administrative, even clinical to clinical, for example. Indeed, vertical integration in an enhanced workflow means that the patient and every bit of information about them accompany each other throughout the entire healthcare process. This is where revolutionary HIT provides tremendous value. While it is up to your organization to choose DIY or work with established software solutions, you will want to do a cost-benefit analysis to determine which is most practical.

Change management for clinical DSS. This is your first transparency. It should lie at the bottom of the stack. More follow in Chapters 10, 11, and 12.

- *Plan every step and test the process.* Since the 1990s, ERP systems software has improved business operational efficiencies while helping to reduce costs. Ask solutions providers to assess your needs to see if ERP will help you implement a streamlined workflow.

- *Organize your skunk works and support teams.* Fill them with great people. Interview many, select few. Obtain commitment and buy-in from each individual; it is essential to change management's successful implementation.

- *Manage your people with interest and compassion.* Assign tasks and responsibilities and continually raise the bar. Give people meaningful work that will engage them. Dale Carnegie said,

"You can make more friends in two months by becoming interested in other people than you can in two years by trying to get people interested in you."

- *Measure.* Be prepared to demonstrate progress and results. Get HIT involved from the outset. Build your own tracking platform and dashboard. You always win when you can visually, graphically represent facts and statistics. Clinical decision support systems are often overlooked, yet they are an effective resource available for implementation from HIT. CDSSs do exactly what their name implies: data-assisted help in decision-making. Although the term *decision support system* is somewhat dated, it still accurately describes a useful tool and component in developing a workflow process.

- *Leadership has changed.* But all too often, the leaders have not. Be a leader and appoint others to leadership positions. Use the character of the people and the accomplishments of your skunk works to demonstrate your CM strategy when presenting it for C-suite buy-in. One change-driven leader is Ford's Jim Farley as CEO in 2020. He claims the Japanese business term *Kaizen* (continuous improvement) as his management mantra. He is also a leader who has recognized how leadership has changed and must continue to change; he refers to his trusted advisors as his "pit crew." None are board members.

- *Communicate, train, and support.* Communicate, train, and support. This is not the only task for your people, so keep them constantly informed and in the loop. Meet regularly, socialize, drop in.

- *Assure you are conforming to all the regulatory rules and regulations.* This aspect of the process must assure that all the procedures and practices connected to change management planning and implementing comply with norms, best practices, standards, corporate culture, and regulations. There are industry standards, internal business standards, and IT standards, as well as your organization's business practices and behavioral and safety expectations. There is governance compliance and state and federal certifications. There are levels of performance and conformance expected by the financial community. All these must be taken into consideration with organizational changes. HIT, with its focus on system reliability, performance, and measurability, is a steady, guiding hand through these dangerous seas.

- *Implement and announce.* Give your change management initiative a branded title and develop it as a continuous improvement methodology. Promote it whenever and however you can. Get people excited enough to help make it work. When you have achieved success, announce internally on Slack then publish articles, give a TED Talk, share on LinkedIn and other social media.

Change management may, at first, seem at odds with all this restructuring and conformance. After all, are we not intending to shake things up? The fact is, with good strategies and standards already implemented and in place, managing change becomes easier to accomplish. For skunk works leadership, there is much value from delivering change management initiatives through the EHR, the CDSS, and other clinical systems.

For clinicians, who might need more "what happens next?" the decision-support software can serve as a computer-based medical consultant. A CDSS integrated into the clinical workflow within the EHR helps deliver desirable outcomes. Many CDSSs leverage expert systems, machine learning, and embedded guidelines and clinical content for just that purpose, and more.

And bear in mind, I am not advocating for an "out with the old and in with the new" overhaul. There are many fine aspects to yesterday's healthcare that ought to be integrated into the new fabric: the seven steps of the Donabedian Model come readily to mind. It is simply that service lines have to give way to deeper clinical process integration; for this, consider using a methodology, either mine or another. Using service lines is like using a folding paper map from the gas station to find your way to your destination. Today's integrated process-oriented healthcare needs to be likened to using GPS mapping on your smartphone, which not only finds the best route but continually updates to steer you clear of traffic congestion.

In all your change management initiatives, always follow the carpenter's rule: measure twice, cut once. In other words, review your quality, safety, access, and anticipated outcomes with your people first to assure you are on the right track. It need not be perfect; you can always make mid-course corrections as needed. But it should already bear the signs of a continuous, change-management, progression.

The RHIT Interview: Ron Wyatt, MD, Vice President and Patient Safety Officer, MCIC Vermont, Burlington, Vermont

1. What was the most significant event or factor that determined your pursuing a career in healthcare?

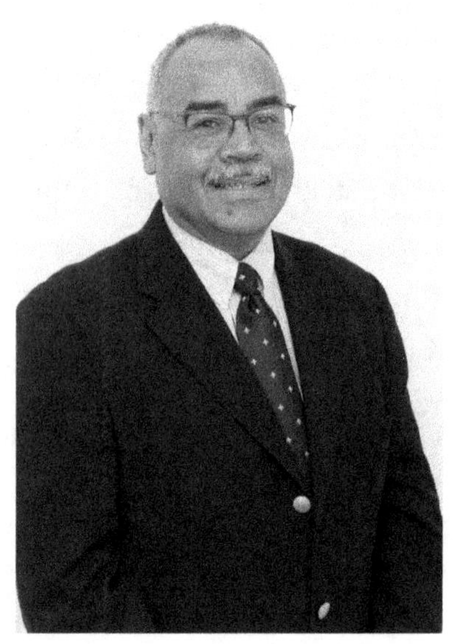

Oh, I could be real brief: racism.

I grew up in rural Alabama, the segregated South. When I was a child, our GP was about sixty miles away. The waiting room was segregated and Black people couldn't even get an appointment. The doctor had a Black assistant who would move the stethoscope around for him. So experiences like these made me look at becoming a physician.

Against all odds, I went to the University of Alabama. When I said I was pre-med, the guy laughed out loud and said, "No way." The math teacher said, "If you can state and prove the Pythagorean theorem, I'll give you an A and you don't have to come back." So I did.

That's kind of why I went into all that. I had decided the best way I could help Black people was to be a physician.

2. After the pandemic is brought under control, what changes do you expect to see appearing in healthcare?

An acceleration of telecare is going to be the main thing. I think a heightened sense of inequities and what to do about them [will drive it] as primarily bigger health systems have to reckon with their past failures that the pandemic has exposed. It goes beyond race, ethnicity, sexual orientation, and gender identity. It goes to rural poor and rural white elderly poor. How can we equitably distribute [clinical] resources to people and populations that don't have access to the internet?

These are just my hopes. I don't know what the hell is going to happen, but it goes back to resource allocation. "Hope" is not a plan, but I do hope that executive leaders will begin to listen, and look at ways to deconstruct how we have always done things. The bureaucracies cannot keep pace with the COVID-19 crisis. Maybe someone will recognize that we don't need all these committees and task forces and work groups to get things done, right? That we can innovate in a much more rapid fashion. Rapid learning cycles.

3. What do you think are the most significant problems facing professionals working in healthcare?

When I'm in conversations, you would almost think Epic and Cerner were actually human beings: if Cerner and Epic can't do it, it can't be done. But they are not like people; they are ways to think about this work in a social-technical environment that will lead to less burnout.

The other thing that concerns me is moral distress as it relates to trainees, which is a type of burnout also. They encounter others who have somehow lost their way. We need to revisit who is admitted in the first place.

Within thirty years this country will not be a majority white nation. Black physicians in the U.S. make up a little less than 5 percent. It was a little less than 5 percent in 1899. The majority of those physicians are in primary care, and many of them work in low-income Black and minority communities, where they lack the resources to provide for their patients.

4. What are the top three reasons you continue to work in healthcare, and how might that change in the next two, five, or ten years?

The top answer is it's just fun. I enjoy it. When I stop enjoying it and it isn't fun, I will stop. The second is to be a role model and mentor younger people. That's not a racial or ethnic thing. I try to provide a different set of thoughts for younger physicians. The third reason is to make some sort of impact on healthcare professionals.

I teach a class on safety, quality, and health policy for the UAB School of Health Professions. It's an interdisciplinary group, for me to share what I've been blessed with in terms of knowledge, and to learn myself. Hopefully I learn something every day.

5. How would you suggest improving and reforming healthcare?

So my first answer is to take out the self-interest. Second, I think the way forward is a single payer universal healthcare system that does not rely on a person's ability to pay, whatever that might look like. Third, we really need to embrace technology, but assure it is applied in a fair and equitable way.

I'm sure you know the stories about the algorithms; the AI, robotics, machine learning, genetic therapies. I'm an old guy, but that is the future of medicine. The pandemic and telecare have pulled the curtain back. The stethoscope is almost obsolete, right? I think those are the things that we'll need to start thinking about—how we are going to embrace those again in a fair and equitable manner.

CHAPTER 10

Applied Change Management and Clinical Workflow

"Workflow is more than just an approach to managing change. It is also a specific set of methodologies and technologies that represent a massive swing in the tools and methods used to support a business process."

—Thomas M. Koulopoulos, *The Workflow Imperative*

Collectively, these four business concepts or practices—applied change management, workflow, information technology, and business processes—are inseparable, deeply entwined functions of the contemporary organization, regardless of the industry. Who among us would not like to see things running more efficiently, delivering ever higher quality healthcare, and fair and just costs for our patients?

Each of the four represent how some aspect of how we think about doing our work, subsequently how we go about using them to improve our work, and by extension our organization. Of course, the computer is the driver for all of them, because it alone has made them feasible. Computers are thinker tools that have replaced nineteenth- and twentieth-century mechanized tools and processes. It is quite impossible to imagine how we could get along without our information-age computers and networks. Both were revolutionary advances that have changed everything about how we human beings live and work.

For us in healthcare, the main reason to implement change management is to improve clinical, as well as administrative, business processes, because "improving quality, enhancing access, obtaining better outcomes, and lowering costs" is the mantra we are expected to chant. When endowed with revolutionary HIT software system tools and processes, the result of this amalgamation is a sophisticated workflow. Once these systems have been developed, tested, and implemented by our HIT organization, productivity accrues from improved workflow and business processes increase. They really must collaborate together.

Some clinicians believe there is no way to surmount the rather disorderliness of today's healthcare system. That is not true. The service lines prove it is correct to attempt better organization. But implementing order is more efficient when it is based on a methodology. The result is a more practical, logically structured workflow, designed and built in partnership with HIT. The methodological foundation helps us understand and tame randomness and chaos, both of which are much in need of resolve in both clinical and administrative business processes. Improving purpose, clarity, and order delivers a sense of well-being and job satisfaction for healthcare workers. This goal cannot be overstated.

What Is Workflow?

There is nothing particularly new about the idea of workflow. People have continually tried to organize their work into meaningful, logical, efficient patterns to improve task completion from time immemorial. Yet our perception and implementation of workflow changed dramatically near the end of the twentieth century. Why? Because of computers and their ability to organize workflows in a far more logical and efficient manner than any former means of automation. Some credit the futurist Marshall McLuhan with predicting the "Information Age" in 1966. It is no secret that computer technology was developed to undertake functions once ascribed only to the human brain, and it has done an admirable job of doing so.

Futurist and author Thomas M. Koulopoulos, quoted above, literally wrote the book on workflow, *The Workflow Imperative*, published in 1995. He defined workflow as a set of human analytical tools, combined with computer-based software tools, that transformed a white-collar work environment into an information factory:

> Or more specifically, a process factory. The process, which can exist in a range of formats from paper to electronic form, provides the basic raw material of every office task. The connection of these office tasks creates a value chain that spans internal and external task boundaries. In this architecture, workflow attempts to streamline the components of the document factory by eliminating unnecessary tasks, thereby saving time, effort, and costs associated with the performance of those tasks and automating the remaining tasks that are necessary to a process.

In other words, workflow, as a computer-aided process for knowledge workers, achieves our goals of better organizing and streamlining task performance, while improving outcomes and reducing costs.

Early automation. Early attempts at automation were often problematic because humans despised operating machines all the day long (and long they were, at least twelve hours). In the nineteenth century, European factories provided free beer to calm and entice workers. Meanwhile, French factory workers protested working conditions by kicking their sabots—wooden shoes—into machines, giving rise to the term *sabotage.* In America, Ransom Olds, the American automotive innovator, built his Oldsmobile Curved Dash on the first auto assembly line in 1902. It was later adopted by Ford and that launched its spread to other industries. Now, most of this repetitive type of work is performed by computer-controlled robotic arms.

Workflow analysis. An observant outsider may, in some hospital environments, conclude there is no workflow, which unfortunately could be true. The U.S. government's Agency for Healthcare Research and Quality (AHRQ.gov) defines workflow as "a series of steps, frequently performed by different staff members and often dependent on related workflows, that accomplishes a particular task. Workflows represent how work actually gets done, not the protocols that have been established to do the work." I define this as a *task-focused workflow.* It must be digital.

Unless the workflow is both digital *and* ubiquitous in daily use, it is not optimally providing the highest quality of care. Why do I say this? You may feel things are working well, or at least well enough. Digital workflow, whether task-focused or human-focused, as evidenced by Tesla's experience, is decidedly superior. A digitally driven workflow possesses tensile strength and flexibility, both of which are essential to continuous improvement. The best way to learn of the advantages to a workflow is to review your current "this is the way we do things here," or better, start fresh. Create a new chart of the workflow using my methodology. To quote further from the AHRQ, "Workflow mapping is a way of making the invisible 'visible' to a practice so they can look for ways to improve their processes to increase efficiency, reduce errors, and improve outcomes." That is rarely effective if it is on paper or only available to the chief of medicine. A transparency created with graphics or presentation software is far more understandable.

Implementing a workflow project is a good task for the skunk works. Unless there is a formal workflow analysis, it is very difficult to identify the processes and, by extension, improve upon them. Individual, team, and departmental tasks, all integrate into the workflow and make use of HIT assets that are essential in determining clinical outcomes, administrative efficiencies, and where HIT decision support is needed. All three must support each other within the workflow, but with this caveat: the outcome (or multiple staged outcomes, as is commonly the case) must be clearly defined and held to measurable standards of efficiencies and compliance with HIT decision support. Once these steps are focused, the how and where of the revolutionary HIT tools ought to be used to craft the workflow that emerges.

Some workflow advocates recommend mapping a new workflow behind the EHR, then adapting (or re-adapting) the EHR to conform to the workflow. This points to the fact that any workflow project must take into consideration the EHR. What ought to happen in designing the workflow is evaluating the efficacy of the EHR and determining if its purposes need to be brought more sharply into focus, thereby presenting an opportunity to improve upon or reinvent it as well. That makes sense so long as you have established the outcome(s) you wish to achieve. Looking at it this way, it seems as though you are beginning at the end, but only insofar as defining with great clarity what you want your workflow to deliver, then using the EHR and other, best, most revolutionary software tools to accomplish that.

Are you collaborative? A hospital may seem to operate as a collaborative environment, but in truth it is more like an ant farm where it appears everyone is working together, though in fact they are not. Their individual positions (nurse, resident, NP, radiologist, surgeon, lab tech) and their differing tasks dictate the patterns with which they perform their jobs. The tasks may be day-to-day operational, repetitive, rotational, urgently needed, or even sporadically "on-call," but whatever they are, that is how they collaborate within the workflow. For example, say a cyclist is brought in by ambulance after a bicycling accident to have his leg treated for contusions and broken bones. Yet during the resident's examination, the patient begins complaining of severe headaches. The team wonders if the patient has suffered a concussion or head trauma. It may be that this drives new workflows for treating bicycle accidents, which immediately assumes different dimensions. Sometimes the work demands bringing in another team, for example a surgeon or a neurologist, to assess and determine tactics. This is not a rare occurrence. But by having described it in the workflows, it can become a datapoint for future learning—how to perform in similar cases with greater efficiency, lower costs, and better outcomes.

Workflow is often affected by the uncontrollable outside influences such as an oversized patient load, equipment availability, and staff shortages. Even so, when workflow patterns are not well-conceived and -implemented, they tend to produce undesirable outcomes. Clinicians may not be chosen for their expertise or other complementary human factors, but simply because they are the only ones on hand and available. This is the greatest random issue in need of a solution. It will be different for every situation, clinician, and hospital.

More and more attention is being paid to aligning the workforce and managing the workflow. A 2020 survey of U.S. clinicians by the Physicians Foundation found that about 16,000 doctors had closed their offices due to COVID-19, with more planning to do so. Fewer doctors necessarily means fewer nurses as well. Most saw a 25 percent decline in patients making appointments, causing concern that many people are not getting the care they need. Touchpoints typically under consideration include:

- High-level patient-staff engagement, as in some of the patterns just mentioned; who is consistently the best clinician for drug overdoses, C-sections, brain surgery? This needs to be quantified with a best-practices assessment to raise every clinician's performance.

- Assurance that the Hippocratic Code tenets of quality and safety of care, access to care, and achieving quality outcomes are fulfilled in every procedure.

- Managing clinical staffing and labor costs at both ends of the spectrum, from hiring and training new staff to developing retentivity policies to assure experienced clinicians do not burn out or leave the profession for other reasons.

- Creating and sustaining organizational health and resilience.

These are not issues that solely concern clinical. They must be bound into workflow patterns with healthcare administration understanding and supporting the clinical workforce management process, regardless of its inherent ups and downs. Both healthcare administration and clinical need RHIT buy-in to stabilize things, to bring its cool logic to bear in successfully mapping their workflows. This is what they are good at, and they have that valuable third-party perspective (not as the observer, but as the partner and assisting problem-solver) and assure everyone has the right type of access to one another in a timely manner.

The thing about workflow is that everyone must know what their job is and understand how and when it needs to be accomplished. Old-school methods such as training meetings or watching a video are, by and large, ineffective: it is difficult to remember, in the abstract, all the hows and whens from them. Revolutionary HIT can minimize that problem, often by simply giving each team member a tablet loaded with the workflow and process app, which embeds the knowledge in the workflow where it can be easily accessed and used again and again.

Virtual workflow. Knowledge-worker workflow today has reduced automation tedium greatly. Our tasks are nearly always virtual, thanks to computer automation. The idea of systematizing healthcare workflow is often thought difficult if not impossible because each patient's situation is seen as unique, yet the principles of workflow can, and should, still apply. This is where change management steps in, because we must improve our clinical and business processes. We all know this is true.

Bedside Consult: Lawrence Leonard Weed (1923–2017)

I had immense admiration for Larry Weed and his work. How could I not? Larry was, in truth, the inventor of the original electronic medical record (EMR). He single-handedly brought clinical care from the eighteenth century to the twenty-first. Larry Weed introduced computer technology to medicine. We have yet to properly recognize him for his innovation and contribution.

Larry was a doctor, a researcher, and an academic, which collectively may have developed his interest in seeking technological solutions to healthcare problems. Healthcare professionals had joked for years and years about how difficult it was to read the doctor's handwriting on a patient record. He saw this pen-and-paper method of recording the interaction between doctor and patient as a problem and was desperate to find a better way. Besides, the handwritten records were categorized by procedures and interventions—physician notes, lab work, X-rays, and so forth. Larry's model restructured it in conformance with a carefully prepared list and description of the patient's medical problems.

The electronic medical record Larry created, introduced in 1964, he termed the problem-oriented medical record (POMR); we now call this the SOAP note, and it soon became the standard. Its progenitor is the EHR, and it led to hundreds of individual software developers creating EHR apps. He trumpeted his new concept in the medical journals and presentations at conferences. He wrote the book, as it is said: *Medical Records, Medical Education, and Patient Care: The problem-oriented record as a basic tool* (1970).

Larry continued innovating. He was instrumental in developing PROMIS in 1970, a computer-based medical information system that deployed the POMR. Its use led to the refinement and widespread use of the EMR, in large part because it employed a touch screen.

His last book—*Medicine in Denial*—which he coauthored with his son Lincoln, was a home run, in which he vociferously claimed that the two things missing from healthcare were standards of care for managing clinical information and electronic information tools designed to implement those standards. It was published in 2011. The conditions it described still exist today, ten years on.

Lawrence Leonard Weed passed away in 2017 at ninety-three years of age. In his lifetime, he was given several awards from organizations you likely have never heard of. Larry Weed should have been awarded the Nobel Prize in Medicine.

Clinical and administrative workflow. You will note the emphasis in this chapter is on clinical workflow. This is quite intentional. In some healthcare organizations, the business process emphasis has shifted from clinical to administrative, due in large part to the massive, complex accounting functions of the healthcare business.

I will defer comment on the arguable political aspects, but will say that there is something fundamentally flawed about the healthcare industry allowing financial decisions rather than science to drive patient care.

Administration is important, indeed essential, but should always serve clinical. Too often, the doctors, nurses, and clinical staff are utterly unaware of anything having to do with patient co-pays, insurer policy benefits, budgetary restrictions, or other administrative rules and regulations that change annually. Too often, patients are admitted for care knowing little if anything about its costs to them or society. We cannot be indifferent to the cost of care. Even pharmacies warn patients of high-priced prescriptions.

These issues, among many other examples, point to the absence of a properly configured workflow. It is certainly difficult to determine how to master so many functions, variables, and problems, but I am convinced they can be addressed when the clinical and the administrative are integrated with one another in a more efficient, impactful workflow, created with a revolutionary HIT system. Once such a system is defined and characterized, particularly in a visual representation (what Mr. Koulopoulos refers to as a value chain), it is easy to spot things that need to change. In point of fact, it is very similar to the use of imaging when preparing for a surgery.

It took Canada fifty years to deploy its universal healthcare system. Perhaps the backlash from COVID-19 will accelerate the changes we must have for healthcare in order to reinvent itself. Will we find that a country such as Finland has experienced higher economic growth because of its COVID containment? Will we see nations such as the South Africa collapse because they cannot get COVID under control? These questions need to be asked, but for now cannot be answered. The pandemic of 2020 was awful, but it also gave us a chance to think about everything we needed to change. Even as we continue to struggle with COVID-19, we are still delivering a respectfully high level of healthcare outcomes, not only for the virus but in our other medical duties. We must constantly reaffirm our commitment to quality healthcare, disregarding the "bottom line." For if we do not refocus on providing quality healthcare, then we will continue to have the same problems with our bottom line. There will be something to bill for, but it will have little value as an outcome.

Capacity Planning

These four chapters in Part III represent our most urgent priorities. As change agents, we must get to work on these matters right now, because defining and implementing a workflow schema will not happen in a day or a week or a month. There are too many people involved, and consensus is imperative. The end result must be explicitly identified first, as mentioned earlier, followed by developing the workflow strategy and selecting the implementation tools needed to begin the change management workflow initiative as soon as possible. Whatever could ease the stress and workload of the clinicians' participation must be taken into consideration. The COVID-19 pandemic had many healthcare people working seven days a week for months on end, with no surcease in sight. At some point the human system breaks down because there is no flexibility or surcease built into the system. When the clinician experiences illness, supply shortages, or even restricted access to food, water, or sleep, it is difficult to have concern for others. In such instances, a hand-wringing HR complaint can be turned into an opportunity for a revolutionary HIT capacity management solution, which is well defined and proven.

How many healthcare facilities can operate at 100 percent capacity or greater on a daily basis? Not many. Perhaps none. But wise capacity planning can accommodate surges in healthcare needs, such as COVID-19 or a natural disaster. Flexibility in capacity planning is essential, all of the time. You cannot adjust to accommodate when you are running at 100 percent. A sensible capacity plan was implemented in New York State by Governor Andrew Cuomo in early 2020. When it was learned they would need twice as many beds as they had, Cuomo asserted bed capacity would be held at 70 percent to accommodate any influxes of COVID-19 patients.

Working with the RAND Corporation, the U.S. armed forces has managed its operations, from peacetime to conflict and back, again and again, using capacity management principles successfully for decades. Mission-critical personnel work staggered schedules that permit periods of "R & R" between duty shifts to help decrease stress. Attrition is considered a solvable problem. So is pilot retention, technical training, and developing innovative treatments for psychological health and PTSD. What can we, in healthcare, learn from the military?

Change management for workflow. The bulleted transparency below was introduced in Chapter 9, and here is the second layer to begin working on. It is likely your organization has separate, distinct workgroups. It is in your best interests to determine if they can be dismantled and reconfigured into pliable, un-kinkable workflows. You may have a workflow of sorts already that needs attention to detail and finessing. Even so, it may be best to simply start from scratch.

- *Plan every step thoughtfully with your core of support teammates.* The attention you pay to detail in the planning phase will reap plentifully as you progress. Use a planning tool or brainstorming so that you get every last speck of detail fleshed out and accounted for. Many are object-oriented so you can design with icons; many integrate with other mainstream software solutions; most have a test-drive option. Then run a visual simulation to test the workflow. Get HIT to help you with this. A virtual test drive will show you how data moves in the workflow and, with HIT's ingenuity, can make it transformative.

- *Once you have a tested simulation, share it with your skunk works team.* You need their suggestions and enthusiasm to move forward, because this is a big change and will require several levels of employee and management participation and support. This includes the CIO/CMIO as a support witness.

- *Manage your people.* Assign tasks and responsibilities to begin the change management effort and attendant introduction of the new system. Implement immediately. Do not be concerned about launching a "big bang" introduction to the new system with, of course, thorough training to accompany it.

- *Measure.* Be prepared to demonstrate progress and results when the skunk works feels it is time. Seek out opinions and suggested best practices from HIT and other institutions. Invite the CIO/CMIO to a meeting and demo it (do not forget to give "it" a name). Deploy IT tools such as a dashboard to give you the analytics you need.

- *Offer to enjoin the CIO/CMIO to lead the change.* Assure they will convey the plan to the rest of the C-suite. Ask for volunteers from the skunk works to begin putting the plan into action.

- *Communicate, train, and support, then communicate, train, and support some more.* Think of yourself as the officer-in-charge of change, leading your troops into what will likely be a jungle of opinion. While you are acting as an emissary for the changes sought, remember to take the feelings and thoughts of the other individuals into consideration or, as Dale Carnegie said, "The only way on earth to influence the other fellow is to talk about what he wants and show him how to get it."

- *Prepare for the long haul.* Just because you have a strategy does not mean circumstances will remain the same, because they will not. Create backup plans, alternative plans, and scenario-specific plans out at least three years so you will not be caught flat-footed.

- *Did I mention giving your change management initiative a name?* Assure your troops, in and out of staff meetings, that this is a continuous improvement project, and that they can participate in shaping it. Little steps, with their help, will lead to big improvements.

For our third chapter and transparency, we take a look at these bulleted change management principles as they apply to clinicians.

The RHIT Interview: Joseph Restuccia, PhD, MPH, Professor of Healthcare and Operations Management, Questrom School of Business at Boston University, Boston, Massachusetts, and Università Bocconi, Milan, Italy

1. What was the most significant event or factor that determined your pursuing an academic career focused on healthcare?

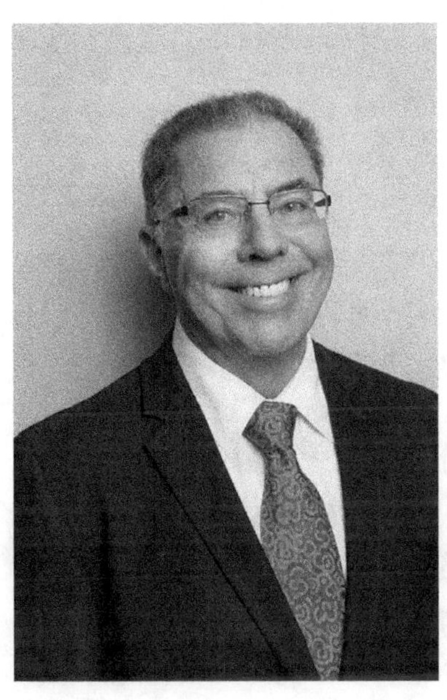

The main reason was that, after college, I had no plan. Well, I did have a plan, which was to be a research assistant to one of my professors, but his grant fell through. So I found myself in June with nothing; no graduate school and no job. I eventually found a job in a small hospital working with the administrator and the hospital's CEO—and really liked it. I knew, if I was to get anywhere in this field, I needed to attend graduate school. I was visiting my brother, who at the time lived near San Jose, and I thought: I'd love to go to UC Berkeley. I applied and there I was, a hippie at Berkeley. It was very, very cool.

2. After the pandemic is brought under control, what changes do you expect to see appearing in healthcare?

There is going to be a combination of expectation and hope. What I do think will happen is there'll be more understanding about the importance of public health. And more resources will be spent on public health, including pandemic control, and in many other ways as well. Part of it will be increasing emphasis on universal healthcare, and whether it comes through the extension of Obamacare—or not.

National health insurance. Medicare for all. I really think that's going to happen. I also think we'll see much more use of technology, which has helped us during the pandemic, particularly telehealth.

As for whether we will see universal health coverage, like the UK's NHS or like Canada or other European countries, I think more like a semi-private hybrid model, like Germany or Switzerland. Although I think it [universal] could be very beneficial, I don't think politically it will ever happen in the U.S.

3. What do you think are the most significant problems facing professionals working in healthcare?

Well, one is burnout. People [clinicians] get very dissatisfied with their jobs. They're placed in no-win situations. A very good example is our fee-for-service system. We pay people on the basis of quantity rather than quality. That frustrates physicians, nurses, and therapists who only want to do a good job and help people, while the system is mission-driven for profit. I expect to see more payment organizations, including Medicare and Medicaid, Blue Cross, United Healthcare, etc., to see that value-based is to their advantage. A win for the provider and a win for the patient. In the long run, costs will be reduced, and it is more holistic, not just for physicians, but nurses too. Perhaps not so much with, say, a physical therapist. There's a Second-Order Effect, but it's certainly something they feel because they're there.

They're measured on the basis of "productivity," which is just as quantitative as for physicians. Nurses feel the pressure, for example the nurse-patient ratio, to take care of more patients as a result of being more "cost-efficient," but not cost-effective.

4. What are the top three reasons you continue to work in health-care, and how might that change in the next two, five, or ten years?

Healthcare is challenging. I love the intellectual challenge. It's possible to both help people do well and to do good. Although I'm retiring from Boston University, I plan to continue to work on a less intensive scale and do more teaching and research. I want to develop and run systems that will support physicians, nurses, and therapists in doing the care they want to do. I want to improve patient outcomes without the financial pressures.

5. How would you suggest improving and reforming healthcare?

Well, I'd say the first thing is universal health coverage. It's absolutely necessary. We see this with the pandemic; people who are working, getting infected, infecting others. With universal healthcare, they could get COVID-19 tests and treatment without worrying about payment or infecting family, friends, and neighbors.

So that's one thing. Another is I think we need to become less dependent on institutional care. We have to provide more ambulatory and home care. There's been a trend in this direction, but it needs to move further towards providing care where people are, rather than where the providers and healthcare organizations are. That could be in the home. We should try to minimize the care that's provided in institutions such as hospitals and nursing homes and maximize care in other locations. And that includes teaching people how to care for themselves with the help of information technology as well as education. We need to move the technology and the providers of care individual providers of care more into being able to provide that care in settings where people live, and particularly at their work or office. Telehealth is a part of that—a very big part of it.

CHAPTER 11

Applied Change Management and the Clinician

"Despite myself, the [$]750 million brings back the Fat
Man and us in Man's 4th Best Hospital at that grave
tipping point when medical care could go one way or
the other, either toward humane care or toward money
and screens—which means money and money ushering
in the decline and fall of all I cared about as a doctor."

—Samuel Shem, *Man's 4th Best Hospital*

Most clinicians would concur: the less change, the better. Yet
everything changes, all the time, and particularly changes in clinical
personnel—in other words, employee turnover—is a nightmare. At
the time of this writing, clinical turnover was rising; various studies
report the annual 18 percent turnover of years past has spiked in
many countries to as high as 44 percent. Nobody, nobody, is happy
about this. Yet clinician staffing is becoming an ever-greater head-
ache and heartache. The trend is not encouraging:

- There is an acknowledged shortage of doctors, increased demand for clinicians, not enough new medical school graduates, and physicians leaving the profession because they are burning out.

- Many hospital clinicians are overloaded with elderly patients (Shem's "gomers"), so they spend their days much closer to death than life.

- A recent U.S. National Institutes of Health study reported, "Physicians who used EHRs reported feeling less satisfied with the amount of time they spent on clerical tasks. They were also found to be at higher risk of professional burnout."

- The shortage of doctors in the U.S. is estimated to reach between 40,000 and 122,000 physicians by 2030. In Romania, the estimate is losing 10 percent over the next fifteen years. In Italy, the number will drop by almost 35,000 by 2028. In Japan, an aging society, the 120,000 shortfall is more than a third of what will be needed.

- Percentage-wise, a concomitant nursing shortage is also impacting healthcare, for the same reasons as with doctors.

- The pandemic's burden on healthcare workers accelerated the number of clinicians leaving the profession due to burnout, post-traumatic-stress (PTSD), and death.

It seems the profession in toto feels overworked, while many suffer from disparities in pay. This is not only an unsustainable condition, it is also intolerable. It is possible the COVID-19 pandemic has caused many to shun a career in healthcare. If young people know what is happening and why so many doctors and nurses are leaving the profession, how can we hope to attract new people—and make up for the growing deficit? We, our society, should not be penalizing clinicians with an onerous burden of debt once they graduate.

Bedside Consult: An Interview with "M," a Pre-Med Student

As clinicians, we need to extend empathy to our patients and ourselves, even more so now as we continue to deal with the COVID pandemic and life becomes ever more stressful. Our empathy must set an example of faith and confidence within our profession, while imparting trust to our patients. Without our optimism, why would a young person want to become a clinician? The road is long and steep, fraught with all the problems of life along the way. Here is the story of "M," a brave young woman who has suffered from serial illnesses since she was a child, all the while sustaining a faith in medicine and the conviction to become a caregiver herself.

"M" is twenty-six years old and has wanted to be a doctor since she was nine. Her interest was due in part to her illness, which began with autoimmune disease and led to others such as vesicoureteral reflux, gastroparesis, and rheumatoid arthritis. She was often quite ill and in considerable pain and trauma, which led to over twenty medical interventions. Although her parents took her to many doctors, none could diagnose the root cause or relieve her symptoms. Yet when she entered college, she was examined by several doctors in the university's medical center. "They were really interested," she recalls. "They were trying to figure everything out and they listened." Over a period of eight years, they were able to treat her to some extent.

M earned her undergraduate degree in health sciences and took an interest in physiology, "especially disease and how it connects to the body. That's what interested me the most." She has seen a number of doctors in the intervening years and comments, "Especially with other issues I've had, the doctor will be in the room for like ten minutes and say, 'Okay, well, let me know how it goes.' You know, as if this meant something and helped."

She is working in a pharmacy as a licensed tech filling pre-scriptions, while studying for her MCAT for admittance to medical school. She is immersed in organic chemistry and, due to COVID, her continuing education is being conducted online. Once in med school, she anticipates she will be studying for perhaps a decade.

M ended our interview with this comment: "I think, like, a lot of doctors tend to think they know what's best for their patients. They're more educated, so they know what's going on. But I think a lot of the times people know when something's wrong with their own body, like, you know, when something isn't right. So I think they don't listen to the patient enough. Once I am practicing med-icine, that is exactly what I will do."

Clinician Workload: Problems and Solutions

Yes, the clinician's day-to-day workload is a large problem. Yes, there are solutions. Doctors and nurses have demonstrated their loyalty to the profession and a willingness to accept a range of workplace disadvantages, some of which were described above. Yet they continue to do their jobs because they are committed to preserving health and saving lives while often risking—even los-ing—their own. Most of us find it difficult to grasp the perva-siveness of patient death, or its psychological impact on ourselves and other clinicians. The pandemic is an international crisis, the likes of which we inhabitants of planet Earth have never witnessed. Healthcare workers cannot be treated as if they were the factory machine operators in Fritz Lang's *Metropolis*. They—we—are the superstar knowledge workers in the aurora borealis of professions: healthcare. Given our superb education; given our commitment to the patient; given the technologically sophisticated technology tools at our disposal—what is the problem?

It may at first seem difficult to identify the problem-solving touchpoints where we can begin changing the cranky, clunky operational aspects of healthcare. Needless to say, there are many such touchpoints. Beginning with people probably makes the most sense: make available to them the revolutionary HIT tools that will instill change behaviors and attitudes, and everything else begins to change behind that. Clinician change must be affected by cherishing and honoring the doctors, nurses, and myriad clinical support specialists who care for the ill and dying. They are doing the best they can and wish nothing harmful to occur on their watch. While this change, and its change management initiative, is a grassroots task, it is best undertaken in small steps. There is no reason why we cannot begin to improve working conditions for clinical personnel now, a little at a time, as we change these other things.

No change means no change. First, we must acknowledge that change is essential. We must be the source of that change, each of us a change agent. Then we must share that message, and achieve buy-in for change management in all aspects, from the C-suite to the HR department. To everyone who is involved in recommending and implementing change management. It will take time and constant reinforcement and adjustments, because change is difficult, but it can be done. Its importance cannot be overestimated: we must improve working conditions for our fellow clinicians or we will continue to lose ever more of them, setting off a deeply problematic chain reaction. A good place to begin is by analyzing how our clinicians are managed, as well as how they manage themselves.

Clinical workforce management. An outsider observing hospital operations might have difficulty determining the tasks to which clinical personnel are assigned. We need a more reliable, visual way to identify healthcare workers by their roles, whether departmental, operational, or task-specific. Perhaps an identification system resembling the military's sleeve stripes, lapel insignia, color-coded name tags, or shoulder patches would be helpful in identifying, recognizing, and rewarding individual clinical knowledge workers in our new workflow organization?

The notion may be useful for discerning if there are logical, repeatable, sustainable people patterns in the workflow: shift changes, time of rounds, even why six nurses are having a well-deserved coffee break at the same time, how long it takes for a doctor to respond to a page, updates to EHRs, and prompt delivery of lab reports, and so on. Although workers are busy and likely doing precisely what they ought to be doing, it may not appear so to the casual observer. This can be due to the randomized nature of the work itself, not the clinicians' manner or behavior in performing it, but this is precisely why television shows seem to prefer showing clinicians in a state of panic and disorder. Perhaps it is what the patient-viewer wants to believe is so. But it is not true at the best hospitals, because the clinicians are driven to provide the best care they possibly can, even if it puts them in jeopardy.

Yet just because it is a broadly accepted media perception does not mean it cannot be changed in practice through an incremental, adaptive change management effort. As recently as the 1980s, some auto manufacturers, when shifting production from one vehicle model to another, did so by dragging the new assembly line templates by hand. Fast-forward to Elon Musk's Tesla assembly line: from 2018 to 2019, it was reinvented from conventional to an "on the fly" production process, almost organic in its ability to adapt to changes. "We believe in rapid evolution," Mr. Musk said in a *New York Times* interview. "It's like, find a way or make a way. If conventional thinking makes your mission impossible, then unconventional thinking is necessary." This observation can, without a doubt, be applied to our healthcare industry. To a great extent, Musk's type of unconventional thinking is promulgated from paying attention to the most minute details, revealed by constant scrutiny of every incremental step, process, and workflow.

Working nine to five. Most patient scheduling is quite out of step with the way our business and social activities work in the twenty-first century. Hospitals conventionally have clinicians working at least an eight-hour shift, but they are not deployed in around-the-clock shifts. A large proportion find they cannot complete all their responsibilities within this time frame and end up working more hours, as many as twelve hours straight, often to the point of exhaustion. Developing an RHIT-driven, more efficient workflow, perhaps around-the-clock staffing, affords the ability to develop complex and intelligent multiple shifts, which makes more sense for both patients and clinical and administrative healthcare personnel. Expansion of service time better leverages fixed assets such as facilities and equipment.

Hospital scheduling can be trying. Some surgeons prefer to operate early in the morning, when they are fresh. Some specialties offer their services only during weekdays, but rarely evenings or weekends. Yet in other occupations, and especially because so many work online from home these days, people rarely adhere to the archaic nine-to-five workday. Life does in fact go on twenty-four/ seven, and so should healthcare. There is little reason why healthcare cannot implement staggered shifts that legitimately go beyond "nine to five," which also obviates overloaded resources and rush-hour traffic both on the roads and in the hospital. Revamped workflows can facilitate these new work patterns,

"Good enough" or best ever? No one questions the devotion of clinicians or their constantly striving to deliver patient satisfaction and the best-ever outcomes. If this is so, how would we respond to a patient being readmitted five days post-discharge for a surgical wound infection after having their gallbladder removed?

Clinical leadership. The best way to interest clinicians in change is to ask them to be a part of it. There are leadership qualities in almost every individual, and by identifying them, and listening to them, change management will be less of an uphill effort. This also applies to the IT members of your skunk works. Let everyone become an expert and a leader in some aspect of your tactics. Eventually, that should extend out to include patients—for example, in focus groups.

Change management for clinicians. Here is the third transparency to aid you in your change management planning.

- *Plan every step and test the hospital process.* Obtain as much information about your existing workflow and processes as possible. If you do not have one, or you are not getting the information you need to make strategic plans and tactical implementations, work with your HIT people to select the best software applications to evaluate.

- *Organize your skunk works and support team.* With the skunk works support and the development of a change management strategy for clinicians, submit your proposal to your C-suite direct report. With their approval, begin enlisting your support team, most of whom have already been identified during the planning step. Now your change management is gathering momentum.

- *Manage your people; assign tasks and responsibilities.* This is the most critical phase: assuring you have a team committed to change. Choose members with demonstrable intelligence and the motivation to drive change. Develop support tools that will keep them informed and involved, such as a KPI dashboard designed specifically to support your skunk works. Involve every member; create milestones and hand out assignments with deadlines. If you give people work to do, and deadlines for accomplishing their work, you can observe your group's progress. Do not forget to manage your own time and set your own goals so that others know you are doing your share.

- *Measure.* Be prepared to demonstrate progress and results. Again, establishing milestones will go far in helping you track your change management. Other forms of tracking and measuring may include or feature an integrated toolset in your revolutionary HIT application portfolio; be sure to use it so you have more than a single perspective.

- *Be a leader and appoint more leaders.* Assure C-suite buy-in. Since scheduling is such a monster, you may need to develop a chain of command unique to your skunk works environment. Assure there is someone at your management level in authority at all times so other members of the skunk works are always informed. Be the leader you want them to be, and appoint more leaders who understand what the group needs from C-suite management and who among them can help get what you need. You are the connective tissue.

- *Communicate, train, and support.* Communicate, train, and support. Constantly. Incessantly. Elon Musk said, "I think it is possible for ordinary people to choose to be extraordinary." Ask others what they need to know, how they would prefer to learn it, then get it for them. Online video conferencing never really caught fire until COVID-19 put the world in quarantine. It has become a nascent revolutionary HIT tool. There are many others, waiting to be discovered.

- *Consider making your change management initiative a branded campaign.* Develop quickie surveys to gain support. Create a website and dashboard just for clinicians where they can get news, ask questions, and communicate privately with one another. Make up buttons they can wear on their uniforms, put up posters, celebrate individuals in any way possible: whatever seems appropriate to instill continuous improvement for the clinical staff, just do it.

So far in Part III, we have discussed applied change management and provided templates for managing your change strategies as they pertain to clinical decision support systems (Chapter 9), clinical workflow (Chapter 10), and the clinician (Chapter 11). Next, in Chapter 12, I present the fourth transparency and will delve into how our change management strategies apply to the most important person in all of healthcare: the patient.

The RHIT Interview: Trent Rosenbloom, MD, MPH, FACMI, Vice Chair for Faculty Affairs and Associate Professor of Biomedical Informatics, Medicine, Pediatrics and the School of Nursing at Vanderbilt University, Nashville, Tennessee

1. What's the most significant event or factor that determined your pursuing a career in healthcare and clinical informatics?

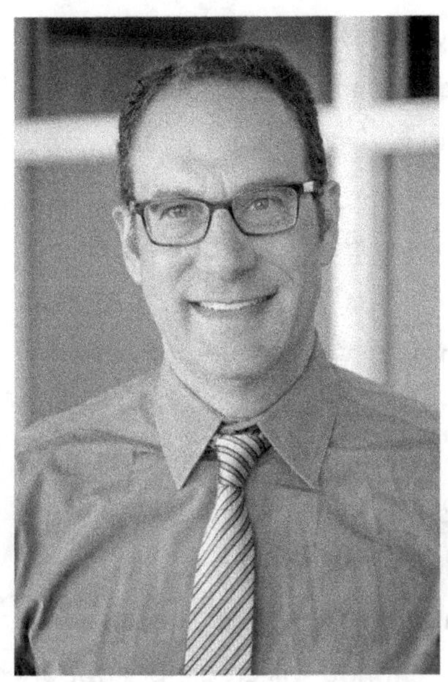

While I was in medical school and residency at Vanderbilt, my initial goal was to become a psychiatrist, but I found that I really loved general internal medicine and pediatrics so I changed my focus. As I was trying to get through my first year of residency, during a rotation in the bone marrow transplant service, I spent eight, nine, ten hours a day writing clinical notes. Then I discovered Vanderbilt's home-grown order entry system had a back door. You could pull lists of meds, labs, and other orders and use them to populate your note-taking template.

Overnight, my documentation went down to an hour or so. Others soon learned about what I was doing, and it quickly became a very popular tool. This experience pulled me into clinical informatics. At the end of my residency, Dr. Randy Miller, the Informatics department chair at the time, offered me a fellowship to continue working in decision support. I took it and I've been in informatics ever since.

2. After the pandemic is brought under control, what changes do you expect to see appearing in healthcare?

What I would like to see is better thinking in terms of technology and policy around alternative approaches to delivering healthcare, including telemedicine and patient portals, apps, and other asynchronous tools. They are really popular with patients and providers, especially during the time of COVID as in-person office visits have declined. Still, these issues are complicated by politics and billing laws. There's this new set of E&M regulations that have just gone into effect, in theory making it easier to document the correct data. You don't have to do all the bean-counting we've done for twenty years when writing clinical notes.

There also needs to be an increased effort to empower patients and put the burden on healthcare providers, and the health system, for all the administrivia. I don't know that COVID has made that better.

Even if the pandemic was to go away tomorrow, we'd still need changes in policy reimbursement practices, and a little more regulation. The updated 21st Century Cures Act will make all clinical data available to patients. That's a great idea, but it needs to be partnered with tools to make it easier for patients to manage their health, wellness, and disease. My hope is that this change will create big opportunities for those developing such tools.

3. What do you think are the most significant problems facing professionals working in healthcare?

A lot of the administrative regulations are burdensome and get in the way of providers caring for patients. Some of the legal frameworks can make patients feel like adversaries rather than partners. It's a difficult time to practice. Right now, the biggest barrier is COVID. It's a really scary time to be on the front lines, which adds to the providers' level of stress. I can only imagine how it adds to burnout as well.

4. What are the top three reasons you continue to work in healthcare, and how might that change in the next two, five, or ten years?

I am around mothers who have just delivered their babies. That's a real high-risk community. I've actually pulled back on doing a lot of the acute care clinical work I have done for years to better focus on aspects of medicine where I can really make a difference. My wife had COVID back in the spring, so the last thing I want is to contract it and pass it on to my household or my patients

Practices will change over the next decade as they move towards telehealth. I know a lot of people in an academic career who have dropped clinical practice, but I'm happy with my work. That could change, but I don't know in what direction.

5. How would you suggest improving and reforming healthcare?

We've been thinking about changes since my early days of clinical documentation, but we have made very little progress. Maybe the government is now listening. Reducing the administrative burdens on clinical documentation. Finding ways to automate or simplify—that would really improve how we deliver care and give providers incentive.

The other area is patient engagement. I don't think we want to put the burden of healthcare delivery and administration onto patients. We need to empower patients to do things they're really good at and take them off of a busy providers' shoulders. Taking medications. Managing symptoms. It's hard to live with asthma, diabetes, COPD heart disease, obesity; but it's even harder if the only "tool" you have is the doctor saying once every six months, "Take your medicine and lose some weight."

There's a lot of evidence of intelligent ways to do this, but not the incentives to bring it into practice. I think that would greatly improve healthcare.

CHAPTER 12

Applied Change Management and the Patient

"Dr. Thomas Dent Mütter (1811–1859): a dazzling, young American surgeon who was so flamboyant and audacious that he wore colorful silk suits to perform surgery, embellished his last name with an umlaut, and was described as the '[P.T.] Barnum of the surgery room.' Mütter was a revolutionary figure whose compassion-based philosophies and innovative surgical ideas and breakthroughs clashed with the constraints of his time."

—Cristin O'Keefe Aptowicz, *Dr. Mutter's Marvels: A True Tale of Intrigue and Innovation at the Dawn of Modern Medicine*

Surgeons in Mütter's time and into the twentieth century were considered rock stars. Another historical figure was William Stewart Halsted, considered by many "the father of modern medicine," emulated in the television series *The Knick*, named after the Knickerbocker Hospital in New York City. Their surgeries were referred to as "amphitheatres" or "circuses," with stadium seating provided so the general public might watch. Often, these spectators would applaud and cheer successful operations.

Where was the patient during these theatrics? Waiting, in some cases without benefit of anesthetic, for the surgeon's knife to cut into their flesh and hoping for a successful outcome. *The Knick* seeks to draw several conclusions. One, Dr. John W. Thackery, the protagonist rock-star surgeon of the series, is a serious cocaine addict, as well as a womanizer of nurses and a blatant, unapologetic racist. His Black antagonist is Dr. Algernon Edwards (a composite character of the two real-life Black surgeons Daniel Hale Williams and Louis T. Wright). Shunned, Dr. Edwards sets up a literal underground hospital, replete with a surgery, in the basement of The Knick to treat the Black patients who are turned away upstairs. Thackery eventually learns he must set his racism aside for the good of the hospital, if not for all of New York City. And he finally has to acknowledge his addiction (cocaine was used as an anesthetic and painkiller at the time, as well as a stimulant in Coca-Cola, and was not outlawed until 1922). The shocker at the end of *The Knick* is how Thackery withdraws from cocaine.

Dr. Marcus Welby Returns

A recent article in *U.S. News and World Report* stated, "In years past, the hospital experience included lengthy stays, severe blind spots in prevention and a lack of patient respect, according to medical historians and health care professionals." It could be said that more recent television series, such as *House* and the long-running *Grey's Anatomy*, have promulgated a grittier healthcare environment and staff than the 1950s' *Marcus Welby, M.D.* For example, as resident doctor Roy Basch in Samuel Shem's novel *The House of God* describes:

I went out into the ward and tried to go see my patients. In my doctor costume, I took my black bag and entered their rooms. With my black bag I came out of their rooms. All was chaos. They were patients and all I knew was in libraries, in print.

Basch is admitting that patients are real people, and he is having trouble dealing with that fact. He acknowledges that his textbook experience is all for naught. Today's patient is, in fact, much more knowledgeable about the practice of medicine—perhaps from watching all those doctor shows on television, Google searches, or YouTube—at least to the point of getting a second opinion. Yet COVID-19 has changed the name of the game: now it is entitled "fake news." There is no pandemic, and even if there were one, I have not contracted it. The doctor's role as a medical authority today is seriously challenged, and it is a big problem.

Yet the next step forward in this relationship, the patient taking a participatory role in determining diagnosis and treatment, is beginning to occur. The proverbial "bedside manner" ought to be participatory, collaborative, and never adversarial. A story is told of a diabetes nurse who snapped at her patient about her irresponsible attitude toward sugar and carbo intake. The patient complained and the nurse was reprimanded.

Bedside Consult: A Patient-Centered Workflow

In the design of successful healthcare information technology implementations, patients matter. Although the importance of addressing the workflow for clinicians cannot be overstated, focusing on patient needs is the new starting point. Knowing how workflow supports and achieves great outcomes helps to ensure that newly designed workflows leverage revolutionary information technology tools. In addition, excellence in workflow design delivers the clinical and financial outcomes healthcare organizations expect. Workflow designers who ignore the needs of patients in configuring HIT-driven workflows can expect to experience either low levels of HIT adoption among clinicians, suboptimal patient care results, and likely both.

The Institute of Healthcare Improvement, led by its founder Don Berwick, MD, who went on to become administrator of the Centers for Medicare & Medicaid Services, displays this mantra throughout its facility:

"Every system is perfectly designed to achieve exactly the results it gets."

Therefore, organizations utilizing new information technologies that mimic the existing clinician workflow deliver outcomes no better than the previous ones. If the workflow is paper-based, the inherent complexity of the information technology in use will assuredly deliver unsatisfactory results. Electronic workflows deliver data and information like a fire hose; a paper workflow throttles that data and information to a trickle of questionable value.

To effectively implement revolutionary HIT, organizations must commit to an in-depth exploration of its greatly expanded capabilities. This impacts not only the practicing clinicians, but must satisfy the anticipated outcomes of all invested stakeholders, from the patient to the CMIO. Readily available healthcare information technologies offer high-productivity tools such as single sign-on (SSO), roaming desktops, location awareness, fast-user switching, and of course dashboards that streamline patient-centered workflows.

Patient-centered workflow, deployed with the RHIT Methodology as its foundation, makes it possible to create a more sensible and productivity-proficient pathway of individual steps. The processes, while remaining distinct, allow for linking and bridging disparate activities, designed specifically for each patient. Even when the workflow is administered by multiple caregivers, the result is superior. Clinicians and IT professionals have created an effective and efficient orchestration of resources designed to enhance both care and cost.

Restaing the Obvious?

It is common to hear "patient-centered healthcare" discussed in clinical circles. Even though it may seem reasonable to say healthcare has always been patient-centered—how could it not be?—we must concede that the morass of administration, financial management, payer reimbursements, all focused on profitability or directed by budgets, has shifted the core of healthcare away from patient concern. Now it is shifting back. That is a good shift, perhaps a tectonic shift in its own right, and we need to refocus ourselves to support it. Here are some of its tenets:

Patients and their families collaborate with the doctor to make important decisions, as opposed to being given a take-it-or-leave-it diagnosis. One of the most puzzling conundrums is how medicine, the purpose of which is entirely on promulgating the healthy lives of patients, could have been so callous toward those selfsame patients. In the past, many clinicians were often brusque with patients, appearing indifferent to illness and its pain and blasé or indifferent to the patient's feelings, whether physical or mental. The portrayal of this indifference went far in *House*: he refused to meet with patients in person. As the series progressed, it was revealed that he had so much compassion for what patients went through (based largely on his own crippling) that he could not stand to see them suffer. Or so the script went.

A 2017 study concluded that in eighteen countries—home to half the world's population—primary care appointments last five minutes or less. Another study revealed physicians spending just over a quarter of their time in patient consults, while nearly half of their time with the EHR and paperwork. Over a quarter of these doctors complained of increased time pressure, stress, and lower job satisfaction. The net is that physicians have been driven to spend less time with patients and more time as an administrative clerk. These issues have not been promulgated by clinicians, but by administrators and payers seeking to increase documentation to substantiate payments. Any time this is the focus, there is no additional benefit accruing to patient care.

Fiscal demands have the effect of turning doctors into commissioned salespeople. For example, compensated telemedicine may adjust some of these policies for the better, and while everyone wants to see clinicians and institutions properly compensated, the patient's health needs to remain uppermost in administering care.

Open notes. Patient data stored in an EHR belongs to no one except the patient, a subject we will return to in Part IV. Full disclosure to the patient—*open notes*—of diagnoses and health prognoses makes all the clinical notes, test results, and pertinent data viewable by the patient. Advanced technology affords the opportunity to display results in interactive visualizations that inform decision-making and deserve to be used more often. Care is not just for physical health, but for the psychological and spiritual well-being of the patient.

Open notes relies on clinical access to database records and the use of revolutionary digital technology to get it into patient hands—and therefore available for patient-physician review. What the patient might think is the doctor's diagnosis and treatment opinion becomes, in digital form, truthful, factual, and accurate.

Equal respect for the values, religious beliefs, and socioeconomic conditions of every patient. All people are concerned about respect for their heritage and are sensitive to prejudice and slights. Clinicians can often slip into favoring those with whom they share a common heritage. In the movie *West Side Story*, Anita sings "Stick to your own kind!" to her sister Maria. That this is a bad idea is expressed in the following scenes. We live in a multicultural society, and healthcare is on its forefront for all peoples.

Fulfillment of the Hippocratic Code between the patient, the healthcare facility, and its clinical staff. The Code embodies a commitment to the highest level of care and safety, praiseworthy access, and the most desirable outcomes for everyone who engages in healthcare, clinician and patient alike. While protected by HIPAA and other government privacy laws such as GDPR, the rules are intended to protect patient privacy.

A century and a half ago, the patient was more or less the doctor's delivery mechanism for the disease or illness. Although that has changed, and no matter how "patient-centered" you or your institution are, the clinician, not the patient, must always be the final arbiter of diagnoses and recommended treatment. But there is no reason the decision-making cannot be shared and discussed with the patient and family. That was not always true, but today it more often is. The pointer has indeed swung from an autocratic treatment method to a collaborative compass point where both patient and physician can become partners in the patient journey.

A century and a half ago, a surgeon did not need to ask permission to perform a hysterectomy or remove an appendix. Today's enlightened patient prefers to know exactly what the doctor has determined ails them and wishes to intelligently discuss treatment options. To decline acknowledging the patient's humanity or even feelings is now considered disrespectful, even unethical. In the movie *The Farewell*, a family unwisely decides not to tell their nana she will soon die of cancer. They discover what a bad decision this is. Patients are consumers. They have choices and know it, and often want a higher degree of control, if not equal participation, while visiting the doctor's office. Even if it flies in the face of the medical diagnosis, the patient has a right to participate in choosing their treatment, even if they decide to decline. But with shifting to sharing control in medical decisions comes more responsibility, which patients likely do not—or would prefer not to—think about. The clinical staff needs to work collaboratively with the patient so both understand what must be done, for example:

- Following through on prescribed care plans,

- Preparing for clinical appointments by gathering essential information for the involved healthcare professionals,

- Routinely exploring the need for second opinions,

- Learning what costs for which patients are liable and comparing prices for medical procedures, ancillary services, or prescriptions, and

- Through dialogue, clearly explaining the treatment plan, and the consequences of non-compliance.

Can the patient be satisfied? Patient satisfaction spans the entire relationship, beginning with entrusting the healthcare system with their health problem, ease of making the appointment, positive encounters with clerical office workers, healthcare assistants, intake nurses, a successful doctor consultation, post-visit paperwork, appointments, and follow-up surveys. This last, asking for feedback on the transaction, should always be followed up by promptly discussing patient concerns about the visit and establishing ongoing regular contact. While all these events may seem self-evident, they are not. They are rarely planned or scheduled, often forgotten in the rush of things, and yet all of them must be completed, as progressive stages in a patient healing/recovery/satisfaction process. They must be consistently and without fail accomplished and documented in the EHR and CRM tools for integral workflow.

Change management for patients. The key takeaways from this chapter, as portrayed in the fourth transparency, are as follows.

- *Plan every step.* Test the relationship and its process. For the clinician, the objective remains always the same, even in the event the patient is recalcitrant like Shem's "gomers." Nobody enjoys being the recipient of bad news, not even the bearer of it. Interestingly, this is where revolutionary healthcare technology can be a help to both parties.

- *Sustain your skunk works and support team at the highest functional level.* Build your clinical team from your best members of the skunk works. Instill trust, respect, and personal allegiance from every person with whom you work. A number of healthcare institutions have come to rely on the concept and its role, even when it is called something different.

- *Continue to manage your people.* Assign tasks and responsibilities. Meet regularly and discuss issues thoroughly. Reach consensus the first time through whenever possible. Assure that every team member is respected, and that their needs are addressed and resolved—again, hopefully right now.

- *Measure.* Continually demonstrate progress and results. Appoint a team member to manage your dashboards—skunk works, its teams, your clinical team and your patients, and ask everyone to use it as if it were a physical meeting.

- *Be a leader and appoint more leaders.* Do as much in teams as possible. Teams may have multiple leaders who can extend their influence outside the specific team. Recognize outstanding work in public ways, for example designating a person of the month on the dashboards. Recognize and develop leadership in others by enlisting their change management skills in the process and outcomes.

- *Communicate, train, and support.* Communicate, train, and support. For example, dashboards and portals are excellent ways to engage and train clinicians and patients in your process. Offer access to a portal or an iteration of the dashboard for patients so they can access both pre- and post-intervention, either on a computer or a smart device. It provides objective evidence and proof, whereas the clinician is often left to verbalize conjecture about what may or may not happen to the patient. Moreover, presenting diagnoses and treatment options via technology—patient educational tools such as clinical articles, websites, or visualizations—in a nonthreatening and non-intimidating manner, portrayed as not just the clinician's opinion but evidence-based clinical diagnosis and treatment outcomes, can be powerfully convincing.

- *Outcomes.* Once you have an established track record with your team and your skunk works, approach your CIO/CMIO or C-suite leader to suggest hospital-wide change management. Develop a list with detailed suggestions for implementations and prepare a presentation to accompany it for wider, higher dissemination. Be prepared to take small steps that allow change to become comfortable for everyone. Give it your all until you succeed.

In Part IV, we come full circle, bringing everything you have read thus far into play to understand how to bring revolutionary healthcare information technology into your organization. You will learn how interoperability is essential to transforming the Hippocratic Code.

The RHIT Interview: André Van Zundert, MD, PhD, FRCA, EDRA, FANZCA, Professor and Chair of Anesthesiology, the University of Queensland, Brisbane, Queensland, Australia

1. What was the most significant event or factor that determined your pursuing a career in healthcare?

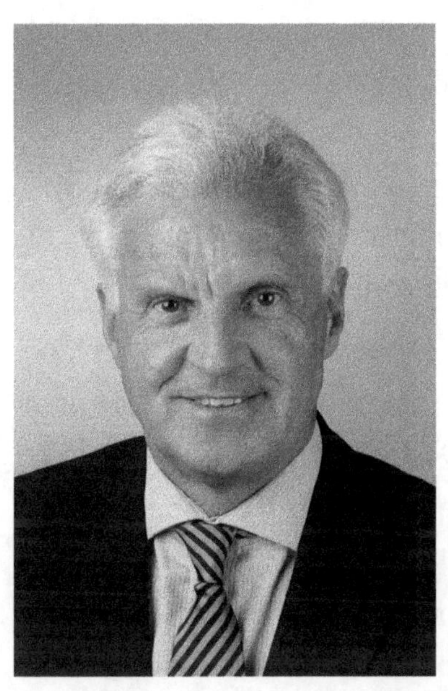

From an early age onwards, I wanted to become a doctor. At age eleven, I wrote an essay explaining I would be a doctor when I was grown up. Our teacher awarded it 10/10 and my "work" was put up on the information board of the classroom as an important reflection paper. By year's end, the sun had completely faded the ink.

I was fascinated by the human body and impressed by the wonderful achievements medical doctors could realize. I wanted to contribute to the relief of patients. I'm a fervent supporter of learning medicine by visualizing problems—"an image is worth a thousand words." In later life, I would advocate Wiki-Anesthesia as the way to teach anesthesia using visual aspects in the big five: teaching, training, testing, quality, and research.

I studied at the University of Leuven, Belgium, and graduated cum laude as a doctor in medicine, surgery, and obstetrics—but I definitively wanted to become an anesthesiologist. I was trained in famous institutions in Belgium, the Netherlands, and the UK, each time focusing on different aspects of anesthesia. For thirty years, I was a staff anesthesiologist at Catharina Hospital, a major teaching hospital in Eindhoven, the Netherlands, until I relocated in September 2013 to Royal Brisbane and Women's Hospital in Brisbane, Queensland, Australia. I have produced over four hundred peer-reviewed original scientific articles—about seventy book chapters altogether. I wrote my first book, Pain Relief and Anesthesia in Obstetrics, together with Harvard professor Gerry Ostheimer, followed by two more major textbooks. The epidural formula which I described in my PhD thesis (1985) is used worldwide as a safe standard for obstetrics (childbirth), gynecology, and surgery. My dream to become a teacher and a doctor were realized.

2. After the pandemic is brought under control, what changes do you expect to see appearing in healthcare?

We often remember wars, but not pandemics. Hence, we have forgotten to be prepared for them; governments lack a plan, and readiness, for the next epidemic. COVID-19 figures are certainly an underreporting of reality. Governments impose restrictions on their people limiting physical contact, but human beings need love and social interactions. As 75 percent of emerging infectious diseases have an animal origin, perhaps we'd better distance ourselves more from animals. The virus has added a new addendum to the ancient Hippocratic Oath to keep our patients from harm: ourselves. Those who pay the highest price, giving their lives to help others, are healthcare workers.

Many say COVID-19 has led to the new normal, but what is that? No stethoscope? No proximity to the patient? How should anesthesiologists examine the airway? How should one intubate in emergency situations? CPR first or PPE first? Daunting questions. Charles Darwin, the proposer of human evolution, once stated: "It is not the strongest of the species that survives, nor the most intelligent; it is the one most adaptable to change." Anesthesiologists [clinicians] have evolved from such calamities in the past and we will rise again, adapting to the new normal.

3. What do you think are the most significant problems facing professionals working in healthcare?

Medical knowledge doubles every eighteen months. Therefore, we need to rethink teaching and education. The Wiki-Anesthesia model could help in providing concise summaries of theories; anesthesia departments need a skillful simulation center, since research is an essential part of our daily practice. All improvements result from research. Without research there is no advancement, and our discipline will go backwards.

We see more and more super-specialization in surgery. Coupled with an increasing cohort of older and fragile patients, who already have more comorbidities, along with a majority being overweight or obese, the challenges for anesthesiologists [clinicians] are enormous.

Therefore, I envision that future colleagues need to make a choice exactly where in the surgical field they'll want to practice.

From a technical point of view, I would be obliged to see ultrasound equipment, readily available in the operating theater to help with inserting central, peripheral and arterial lines, regional anesthesia blocks, and to also evaluate the patient's cardiac condition. Videolaryngoscopy should be the default intubation technique, and vision-guided insertion of supraglottic airway devices should replace the blind insertion method, as more than 50 percent of these are mal-positioned.

4. What are the top three reasons you continue to work in healthcare, and how might that change in the next two, five, or ten years?

I'm passionate about anesthesia: it has been my profession for a very long time and I still enjoy it very much. I work as a team member. I can combine it with education (teaching, simulation, supervising PhD candidates and other higher degree students), research, and lecturing. I'm often asked by international journals to act as a reviewer in the essential peer-review process of manuscripts.

I've never regretted any part of my professional career, and would do it all over again. I am blessed to work with amazing teams and international colleagues on solutions for problems we face in anesthesia.

Not resting on my laurels, I keep on being fascinated by so many challenging aspects of our specialty. Ongoing involvement in research, including major advancements in anesthesia and medicine in general, stimulate me. There are still so many queries that need an answer. And I simply enjoy it.

5. How would you suggest improving and reforming healthcare?

We need to be prepared for the next epidemics and/or pandemics, for surely they will come. The year 2020 proved we were not prepared for COVID-19. Hospitals and Ministries of Health need a plan ready to use for disasters. Specialists need to be informed how to deal with these new infections. Doctors need to learn how to better protect their patients, themselves, and their loved ones.

My suggestions:

- Advancing the quality of care through improvement in acquiring knowledge; we need better techniques with which to teach and study material.

- Access to online simulation in anesthesia and a wide variety of clinical skills.

- Providing transparent data and evaluation on long-term outcomes for surgery patients.

- Using IT-based systems, preferably nationwide, as we need the "big data."

- Improving hospital organizational operations, while focusing on patient and employee well-being; it needs to be an ever-evolving process. Medical information should be transparent and available to the public.

- Improving affordable access to quality healthcare for all people, wherever they may live.

- Providing insurance, public and/or private;

- Engaging patients through education (prevention of diseases); ease of access to patients' files (wherever they are); providing standardized information essential in treating emergency patients and patients' forums.

- Hospital management and human resources to support clinicians and clinical specialists working long hours in physically and emotionally demanding jobs. Quality care for patients can only be provided if hospitals also pay attention to the well-being of their staff.

Part IV

Revolutionary HIT

In the early 1980s, about the time IBM introduced its eponymous Personal Computer, the esteemed weekly computer newsmagazine *Computerworld* published this promotional advertising:

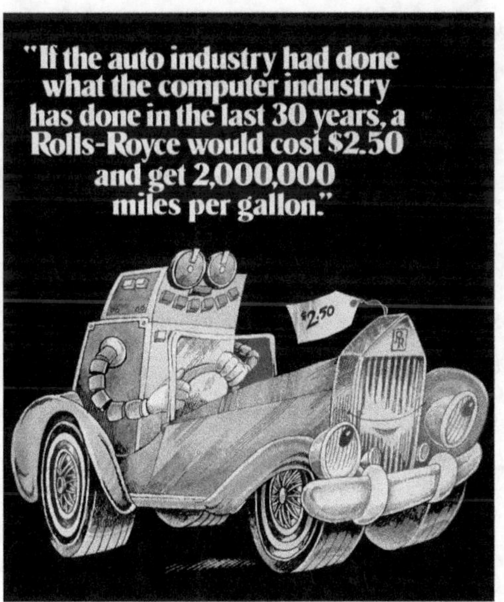

Fast-forward this analogy through time and space to 2021 and a comparison between the automobile and healthcare industries. Might it read something like this?

"If the healthcare industry had done what the automobile industry has done in the last 30 years, we would have a cure for cancer, people would live to at least 120 years of age, and the cost of care would be 50 percent less than it is today."

In the Introduction, I provided you with this definition of revolutionary healthcare information technology:

Revolutionary Healthcare Information Technology (RHIT) offers clinicians, researchers, and administrators immensely powerful tools to drive clinical and administrative processes to deliver high-quality, safe, accessible, and investment-responsible medical outcomes.

In the chapters that follow in Part IV, I reveal the practical application of this definition. The meaning of "revolutionary" will become crystal clear. You will grasp how technology tools and your relationship with the HIT people can create the change essential for the health and well-being of healthcare itself. I will knit together what we have learned thus far into a realistic scenario, baked into my RHIT methodology, in which you will come to understand how a new way of thinking about workflow and process is the means by which these tools, in synergy, can make a difference and make healthcare better, stronger, more efficient, and more satisfying for clinicians, administrators, and patients. In short, healthcare can reach a new level of the Hippocratic Code if you and others who share the vision do the necessary work to make it so.

By all accounts, the healthcare industry has had a couple of metaphorical flat tires. It might even have suffered from an ailing transmission, or perhaps an engine that has run out of motor oil and is clanking its way to ever greater dysfunction. By most accounts, healthcare is stuck, spinning its wheels in the mud of its past.

Look at auto technology. Thirty years ago, the auto industry was pretty much in the same configuration as it had been since Henry Ford's assembly-line days, and the expected life of an auto averaged sixty thousand miles—which is to say the auto industry was in about the same shape as healthcare had been for the same length of time, and still is. But look at autos now; a 2021 vehicle is so well built and reliable that it will operate for two to three times as long as one built thirty years ago: at least two hundred thousand miles. Most autos hardly ever need maintenance beyond an infrequent oil change or software update.

Auto prices and profit margins are rock-bottom, yet cars are bedecked with more and better technological features every year: Wi-Fi, adaptive cruise control, collision avoidance systems. On average, the 2021 vehicle has up to sixty microprocessors and as many as a hundred sensors, most engaged in keeping people safe. Today's auto is so good, in fact, that everyone in America is driving a new or a nearly new car for about ten years, reaching such market saturation that the industry is having a tough time selling those new F-150s year after year...

...or at least vehicles powered by an internal combustion engine.

The battery-powered electric auto changed many more aspects of our world than just the engine under the hood. Its impact on the oil industry is as earthshaking as was the discovery of shale deposits. A few years ago, pundits predicted the emergence of electric cars in 2050, but look what happened: revolutionary technology, much of it driven—if you will allow a pun—by Tesla. Electric cars mean either a decreased or no need for gas refueling stations. Aside from the government tax credit award, they diminish gas tax revenues and, proportionally, funding for highway maintenance. Of course their greatest impact, hopefully, is on lessening many forms of pollution.

To what can we point as the reason for a staid, hundred-plus-year-old industry reinventing itself as the auto industry has been doing?

Technology, of course. Technologies on the factory floor, technologies in the supply chain, from mass-manufacturing to customization, to high-tech logistics for delivery to dealers and customers, and embedded technologies in the car itself.

In 1889, Charles Duell, the commissioner of the U.S. Patent Office, said everything that could ever be invented had already been invented. How shortsighted he was. We had just begun exploring electric technology, removing lamps that burned whale oil from homes and replacing them with light bulbs.

In 1984, Apple introduced the Macintosh computer with a Super Bowl video advertisement, broadcast once only, positioning it against IBM with a vivid analogy to George Orwell's novel *1984*. Everything about the Mac was revolutionary. Innovative. Technologically state-of-the-art. Compared to the Mac, IBM's Personal Computer was as stodgy as a 3270 terminal, and that is pretty much where it has stayed.

In 2020, Chris Deaver, who spent four years in human resources working with Apple's research and development teams, told the *Wall Street Journal*, "This is what most people do not understand: Incremental is revolutionary for Apple. Once they enter a category with a simply elegant solution, they can start charting the course and owning that space. No need to break speed records, just do it organically."

The revolution is happening in every endeavor where the need exists for technological innovation and new "what-if" thinking, from Dan Bricklin to Elon Musk and beyond, to the next revolutionary technological innovator in healthcare.

- Chapter 13 recounts some of the exploits of Elon Musk, a technology visionary worth emulating, then goes on to explore the imagined intersection of innovation, revolution, and technology, pointing healthcare's direction.

- Chapter 14 dives deeply into the intersection to follow the yellow brick road to revolutionary healthcare technology's nirvana, interoperability, which is something of a cautionary tale as subsequent chapters explain.

- Chapter 15 asks the question: When clinicians seek quality of care, is a procedure or intervention ever just "good enough"? How can we know what is good enough and what is revolutionary quality?

- Chapter 16 probes the matter of revolutionary access, the linchpin connecting quality and safety to superior outcomes. Access is often taken for granted, when in fact it has many facets and plays an essential role in delivering revolutionary healthcare.

- Chapter 17 challenges the less-than-precise use of the term *outcomes* in making the case for revolutionary outcomes. The different types of outcomes are described and posited against the higher revolutionary standard, which is what each of us must strive for.

Chapter 13

You Say You Want a HIT Revolution

"If you go back a few hundred years, what we take for granted today would seem like magic—being able to talk to people over long distances, to transmit images, flying, accessing vast amounts of data like an oracle. These are all things that would have been considered magic a few hundred years ago."

—Elon Musk

There is no "one-size-fits-all" implementation of revolutionary HIT. It is not reliant on a single technology—for example, the often-touted "artificial intelligence." It may, or might not, come from the IT department's technologies. Its sole wellspring, or call to action, is always the mind of a human being who thinks there must be a better way. This change of mind may come about through deliberation, while a different awakening may be a scintillating discovery. Both incremental and instantaneous revolutionary HIT are valid. The truly revolutionary thing about the many advances in information technology is that they are self-propagating.

Technology reinvents itself over and over, as evidenced by the "what-if" analysis brilliantly implemented in the Bricklin-Frankston VisiCalc. It gave birth to the term "killer app." It was indeed revolutionary, because this technological what-if tool gave us a new way to think about modeling problems, then quickly and accurately testing various hypotheses. What-if is a thinker toy for innovators.

Bedside Consult: Elon Musk: The Eclectic Entrepreneur

Elon Musk—whether you admire or despise him—is an innovator of the first order who has used technology to change the way Americans engage with the world in many ways.

- Musk's first entrepreneurial venture was the Global Link Information Network, an online city guide, in 1995, with his brother Kimbal and Greg Kouri.

- He used the money from selling Global Link (aka Zip2) to fund the company that would become PayPal, which he sold to eBay. PayPal gave both individuals and businesses an instant, easy-to-use payment system that obviated checking accounts, wire transfers, and often float.

- The sale of PayPal led to Musk's founding SpaceX, a rocket engineering company for launching satellites, International Space Station supplies, and astronauts. One of his most impressive innovations was capturing and reusing rocket modules after launch. The Falcon 9's technological innovations far and away exceed anything built by NASA. Its first stage autonomously lands on the deck of a robotic ship, thereby making it reusable for SpaceX to capture and share detailed data, using a multitude of sensors, to make it safer and more reliable.

- Tesla Motors, an all-electric automobile company, launched in 2003. Its first vehicle, the Roadster, was introduced just five years later. Powered by a lithium-ion battery, it traveled 250 miles on a charge. Since then, Tesla has introduced the Model 2 with autonomous capability; the Model 3, a moderately priced Volkswagen of electric cars; the Cybertruck pickup; and the semi-autonomous Tesla Semi.

- Most recently, Tesla has introduced an innovative, low-cost solar roof and large-capacity storage battery system for homes.

Elon Musk has created a technology-infused revolution in every industry he has touched. Imagine what his kind of thinking could do for healthcare!

When Musk decided to build LI battery-powered, cutting-edge vehicles, he likened Tesla Motors to a personal computer company, not an auto company. Musk envisioned outsourcing a lot of the manufacturing to streamline the value chain, shortening build times but not necessarily lowering costs. He did not get all of that right, but he and his people were nimble enough to change their strategies and decision-making to get the logistics and innovation back inside his own factories. Tesla had a few more bad breaks, but it survived because it saw itself as a key player in the rapidly emerging alternative energy economy. Tesla embraced technological innovation in everything it could, from an all-electric vehicle running on batteries to building a truly autonomous vehicle. Musk even pondered combining SpaceX and Tesla technology to make a flying auto.

The Intersection of Innovation, Revolution, and Technology

Musk's, and perforce Tesla's, accomplishments were the fulfillment of the hopes and dreams of the existing auto industry, against which it continues to struggle. Even so, by deploying many kinds of high-technology innovations—some innovative and others not so much—the result is the reality we all drive every day: high-quality, safe, technologically magnificent, fuel-efficient automobiles at an affordable price. Are there parallels between the auto industry and our own? Are not our objectives similar? What lessons might we learn that would apply in healthcare, which, if we were to study them, might help determine our capabilities and adaptability to change? How do we begin thinking seriously outside our box about managing change?

For Elon Musk, it was to stop thinking of Tesla as an automaker and instead more as a computer company, essentially marrying rapid application development with on-the-fly changes on the assembly line. Musk watched, learned, and determined the ways in which Tesla manufacturing was not going well. Then he thought back to his experience in technology companies and created a what-if model that he thought might solve its problems. If you will permit another automotive analogy, Musk saw himself standing where three thoroughfares met and crossed one another: Innovation Street, Revolution Avenue, and Technology Parkway.

As Tesla built more and different electric vehicles, it created a sea change across all the oceans and land masses of our world. It was Musk's and Tesla's innovation, deployment of revolutionary information technology, and progressive leadership, determined by using what-if analyses to solve its problems and map the route to changing not just auto manufacturing, but the world. I hope this book will inspire you to create and implement this kind of profound change to healthcare. I believe we can learn a great deal about what works and what does not for our industry by studying how other, completely unrelated, industries have outgrown old habits, innovated with revolutionary ideas, and changed to meet the challenges of today and tomorrow. Let us take out our smartphones, open our map guidance app, and take a look at the junction where innovation, revolution, and technology meet.

Innovation Street. What Elon Musk learned is that conventional thinking about technological innovation, as our *Computerworld* poster illustrates, is just that: conventional. Putting out daily fires and being constantly on the edge of chaos is not going to get healthcare situated on the forefront of change. Innovation helps us move away from the conventional and toward revolutionary HIT. It is quite the opposite of the way most think about, and use, information technology. We are in rather desperate need of making fundamentally new, extraordinary changes in how we practice, manage, and dispense healthcare.

The way to understand, analyze, and deploy these changes begins with contemplating how we can innovate. If you are not an innovator, you can develop those skills. Study innovation and innovators, and apply what you discern to your own situation. What would Steve Jobs do in your position? It was he who said, "Innovation distinguishes between a leader and a follower." Take chances. Encourage teammates to define issues and take problem-solving risks. Share your studies and learning with others in the skunk works to promulgate new ways of thinking for everyone. It can be . . . well, contagious. Once you have innovation flowing through the skunk works' veins, it is time to let it flow down Revolution Avenue and throughout the organization.

Revolution Avenue. Gartner Group studies have ascertained that many of the business strategies prior to the COVID-19 pandemic are no longer performing well and need to be rethought. The Gartner recommendation is to perform a "reset" in three phases:

- *Respond*: immediately ensure workers are safe and primary business operations are continuing;

- *Recover*: stay the course and work on a strategic restoration plan that analyzes weaknesses and either eliminates or turns them into strengths; and

- *Renew*: carefully institute the new strategic plan and monitor workflows and processes to assure its success.

This is how it was always supposed to work. Everything we do and create should add value to our mission. When it is not up to snuff, it must be changed. What may have passed by our attention was the fact that this level of revolutionary change could be accomplished in a systemic way that does not pile chaos upon chaos. In many cases the bureaucracy has an "if it isn't broke, it's fine" mindset, or it does not want to spend the time and money to find something better. They must be disabused of this notion, for it is shortsighted and more costly than implementing the innovations so necessary to healthcare's revolution. "Good enough" thinking is an obstacle to doing better—and it is not enough.

Technology Parkway. Innovation and its attendant revolutionary practices get us to the Technology Parkway. Technology is the key in the change management ignition. (If your car is very new, all you may need to do is touch a button.) Every car, accelerating onto the parkway, drives us toward solutions to our dilemma. Your healthcare skunk works and/or team members are, by and large, technologically literate. They understand how to use their everyday software tools, but may not know or understand their advanced capabilities. Software usage analytics can determine if the software applications your knowledge workers use are truly providing revolutionary performance and productivity value. If the results are disappointing, it makes sense to offer more training or perhaps install a new, better software package. Use analytics to identify problem areas and poor processes; then modify those processes, and test them again with analytics. Now, move forward to monitor and identify those that may need rework. If you do not assure that every knowledge worker is data-literate, stretching and extending themselves and their system- and software-acumen every day, then no innovation is occurring, thus no revolutionary new practices, and no new uses for technology. So nothing of any significance will change.

The Road Ahead

Interoperability is our destination on the Technology Parkway. At its core, interoperability is why healthcare sorely needs revolutionary information technology for administration, clinical practice, and for IT itself. Interoperability is often mentioned as a desirable outcome, but it is also healthcare's most difficult garden-hose kink to unsnarl. A great deal of work remains to be done to create a consistently high-performing, truly interoperable enterprise, the subject of our next chapter. That work must be performed by the healthcare institutions, working with the governmental standards and the software vendors to ensure that all the requirements are agreed upon and everyone is intent on achieving interoperability. The healthcare institutions need to press their case and establish goals. The government must continue to put teeth into regulations, such as for preventing data-blocking. Software vendors must recognize that they own the code, but not the data.

The sad truth is, interoperability is not a turnkey task. It cannot be accomplished without continuous attention and refinement. It is going to require a herculean, revolutionary spirit to make the changes that must be made. All three organizations—healthcare administration, clinical practice, and HIT—must do it together, as equal partners with the same goal of interoperability. In so doing, they become transformational. They become revolutionary.

How might that happen? Although there is no one-size-fits-all path, by adapting the Musk/Tesla example to your environment, the work you and your teammates do in your skunk works can produce new paradigms for change. You or another of your leaders might have found a revolutionary technology tool, and the skunk works might indeed be enthusiastic about implementing it. But assure it is not a stand-alone solution to a specific problem. It must be one step in a strategic plan, not a one-off, finger-in-the-dyke fix.

As the next three chapters discuss, your implementation of deploying revolutionary HIT can reap benefits if you follow my RHIT Methodology presented here, with the intent of implementing more efficient workflows based on your new strategic process. The intersection of innovation, revolutionary strategies, and implementing state-of-the-art technology is where your knowledge workers—clinicians, administrative staff, HIT, and patients—can unite to solve problems and work together to achieve a higher level of successful outcomes. Expect to experience turmoil, disruption, resistance, frustration, and, yes, a great deal of change. Be assured it will all turn out for the best. Because it has to.

The RHIT Interview: Carlos Joel Formiga Xavier, Country Manager for MphRx Brazil, São Paulo, Brazil

1. What was the most significant event or factor that determined your pursuing a career in healthcare information technology?

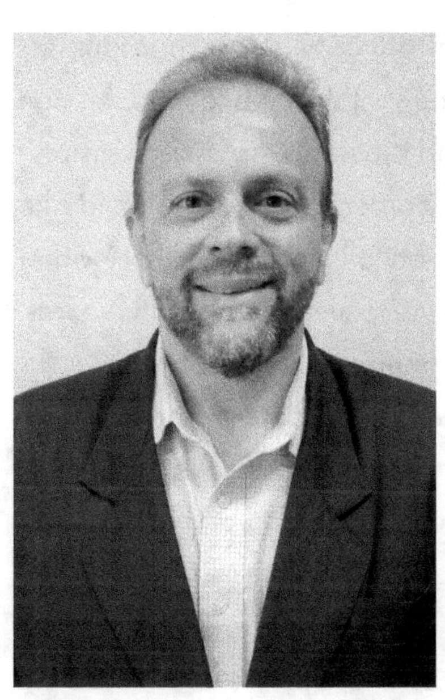

I started in technology as an engineer, developing a sales, then an executive, career at IBM. Towards the end of my twenty-five years with that company, I held the position of Director for Public Sector in Latin America. Smart cities were the tech wave of the time; very promising. That was when I decided to move into government as a second career and to take a master's degree in political science in preparation for it. I came in contact with public health while working as an assistant for the governor of São Paulo, but it wasn't until I engaged in a political campaign that I fully embraced healthcare information technology as my new area of expertise. It became a pillar of the mayoral candidate's campaign program, and I ran it under his administration for the city of São Paulo. As this politician moved up to governor, I went on to run a digital innovation in healthcare program for the largest and richest state in Brazil.

2. After the pandemic is brought under control, what changes do you expect to see appearing in healthcare?

This could be answered in many ways. I am going to focus my answer on health IT and in particular the explosion in tele-consultation caused by the pandemic. I am convinced this is the start (a fast start) of a more profound change. For now, what we witness is a dramatic shift from in-person to video conferencing in caregiving. Probably too much of a swing, and we are likely to see it balance back toward in-person after the pandemic. But the long-term effect, in my opinion, is in the fact that video consultations are digital events, which means scheduling and eligibility are done online, previous history or lab results are accessed digitally, vitals are acquired through remote devices or even camera-based algorithms, prescriptions and (specialist) referrals are done and forwarded digitally. This builds the data infrastructure for digital consultation to emerge from these video events. I see not only a stricter adherence to electronic health records, but also the advancement of digital screening/triage, better integration of patient history, increasing adoption of data-based/digitally implemented care protocols, and maybe more patient engagement via digital access tools. From video consultation to digital care: this is the big impact the pandemic will have on healthcare IT, as I see it.

3. What do you think are the most significant problems facing professionals working in healthcare?

Probably keeping up with the latest in their fields. The speed and volume of medical knowledge is advancing beyond the human capacity to absorb, select, connect, and consolidate with previous knowledge, and then apply it. Not to mention the additional pressure, since patients are more (not necessarily better) informed through "Doctor Google." For the clinicians dealing with the COVID-19 pandemic, this is also true, as studies are released in preliminary stages demanding tougher scrutiny in the midst of fake or incomplete news.

4. What are the top three reasons you continue to work in health-care, and how might that change in the next two, five, or ten years?

Number one is relevance: not just the general idea that working in healthcare is so important to people, but the fact that working in healthcare IT specifically addresses the most significant issues of efficiency and effectiveness in one of the most resource-consuming activities in our economies.

Number two is opportunity: healthcare is one of the least digitally transformed areas of our societies in comparison to any other (logistics, finance, commerce, social media, transportation, etc.). This means there is so much yet to be achieved and the general perception is we are at the right place for change.

And number three is career: there are still very few of us who can talk technology, data, patient diagnosis, and treatment, all in one coherent sentence. We are in high demand. I don't think these three factors will change much in the next two to three years. I would hope, though, that in the five- to ten-year range, a lot of the gain in digitization will have been achieved; there will be more professionals with better structured careers, so opportunities might be less abundant. But healthcare IT is still an attractive work area to enter about now.

5. How would you suggest improving and reforming healthcare?

Allow me to add my perspective in one dimension of this reform: the consolidation and sharing of patient data throughout the continuum of care. Interoperability, in one word. Consolidated or unified health records, in three or four words. This is the holy grail of healthcare IT, and may be of healthcare as a whole, as discontinuity is currently the norm with horrific effects in both efficiency and clinical efficacy. My suggestion is that we bring the patient to this unsolved equation, to act as the broker of his or her own clinical history. This is not just an IT challenge, but a regulatory, institutional, and cultural one. We providers and payers have tried and failed miserably to solve this discontinuity. Governments here and there have made only marginal progress. It is now time to bring those really interested, those who currently pay with their money, their health, or their lives, for this lack of progress: the patients.

Chapter 14

RHIT and Interoperability

"The temptation to form premature theories upon insufficient data is the bane of our profession."

—Sherlock Holmes, *The Valley of Fear*

What every clinician wants is complete and immediate access to clinical and patient information. This is what we in healthcare commonly regard as informatics. A needs analysis, conducted by HIT, will determine how frequently and successfully informatics is providing the best available data at the right time and place. (If you need an example, consider that research posted on websites often does not have a date of publication; you could be reading about research done yesterday or ten or more years ago. Data does not have an expiration date, but information does.)

The fundamental purpose of RHIT is its ability to gather data and extract essential information for people to use in accumulating knowledge. This is what computers and information processing have always been about, ever since ENIAC, the first digital computer, calculated missile trajectories during World War II. We all understand that, and RHIT does a good job with informatics.

So let us be less concerned with informatics and more focused on the eight-hundred-pound gorilla in the room: interoperability. Research points out that across healthcare, interoperability remains a problem in search of a solution. Further research has determined that, compared to acute-care institutions, post-acute facilities' technology implementation lags by ten or more years.

In some businesses, this might be considered "good enough." But it should not and cannot be considered superlative performance in healthcare because human lives are at stake. It speaks to the fact that we think we are working with state-of-the-art technology, but is it true? We often know when our system is not performing at an optimal level. We constantly wonder what we can do about it. We know we need to be on the cutting edge of medical technologies.

Brittany Kaiser, cofounder of Own Your Data Foundation and author of *Targeted*, said in an interview, "Data is the most valuable asset in the world." I would say this is almost correct: the most valuable asset is people, followed by data. No people, no need for data, right? But let us use this assumption to assert that clinicians need more and better data to make more and better decisions on behalf of our patients. What is that gorilla standing in our way?

It is the electronic health record. The EHR is the first and most important data repository in our workflow. Yet obtaining its data to turn into information and then knowledge, and ultimately transform it into a blueprint for patient care, is often a frustrating, clumsy process. How have we allowed this to happen? Some of the issues:

- Data storage has advanced rapidly over the past decade, and methods differ greatly between proprietary computer systems. Many perceive their EHR as little more than a data storage facility, which is unfortunate. No one asks what the problem is, so no one can solve it. There have been extraordinary advances in storage technology, in part due to the every-growing amount of data but also the broader range of data, such as audio, video, streaming, and so forth. Repositories for data storage are often in the petabyte range, and will soon grow to exobytes.

- Computer systems—informatics—have an ever-deteriorating life span. Older single-function stand-alone systems do not get replaced because of the disruption inherent in converting, as well as the cost. Both lead to being stuck with the status quo and not solving deeper informatics-level issues and problems. For example, integrating these older systems with newer, higher-performance ones often cripples both. The result is a lost opportunity to deliver better, faster, less costly solutions.

- According to the Stanford Medicine study of five hundred American doctors, conducted by the Harris Poll, "Seven out of 10 PCPs (67%) think solving interoperability deficiencies should be the top priority for EHRs in the next decade—and 43% want improved predictive analytics to support disease diagnosis, prevention, and population health management." Interoperability software tools can take data from an EHR or from a laboratory system and share it with an administrative system such as billing, accounting, payer-related compensation, or even an admission discharge transfer system. Yet few such tools exist for doing the same thing for clinical purposes because clinical data interoperability is not perceived as a value-add by EHR vendors. As a result, we have allowed the EHR software vendors to have their way with the data they collect. For example, an individual physician's office staff may be using an EHR from the same vendor as the hospital where he practices, but if the versions are different, there is constrained interoperability. The two offices may end up printing the information on paper and faxing documents, in a few instances emailing a PDF, or transmitting an unsatisfactory continuity of care document (CCD).

Interoperability is also the Achilles heel of healthcare, because of the complexity and diversity of its issues, only a few of which you have just read. There are lessons to be learned from this technological awkwardness, missteps and seemingly unresolvable roadblocks. Learning those lessons is preparation for creating interoperability in the healthcare enterprise.

Much of the healthcare industry is hobbled by outdated business practices; we have converted a paper process to a quasi-digital one without taking full advantage of what digital can provide. There are too many moving parts and no desire to coalesce them into seamless workflows, even though there is revolutionary information technology to do so. Our advanced networking capabilities have made sharing information quick and easy, so then why do we balk at taking advantage of this to move our workflows forward? Because change is hard, or so we think. Yet connecting healthcare technologies to create and enhance interoperability is at the heart of the revolution. It is an adventure without an end. It is borne of commitment and resilience and open-systems thinking, and made possible because people talk and work together to make it happen. It is possible if we are willing to cross the bridge while enduring a small amount of pain. We can simply set our eyes upon the new path and make it so.

Bedside Consult: Recent Trends in Interoperability

It is well known and understood that interoperability is critical to delivering quality patient care and transformative outcomes. In the process it ensures better safety of all data made available to caregivers, reduces or obviates duplicate testing, and results in less critical data going missing. I have written in its favor for years and years. It is one of the mountaintops we must scale in implementing RHIT. In that respect, it is either K2 or Everest. But it can, and will, be accomplished.

Although clinical interest in interoperability has languished for year after year, a watershed event occurred in February, 2021: the Office of the National Coordinator (ONC.gov) released its latest Interoperability Standards Advisory (ISA), reference edition. This is the most comprehensive overview of interoperability implementation since 2014 in the Health Level 7 (HL7) C-CDA standard, which was, sadly, largely ignored by EHR software vendors, who perceived no economic benefit accruing from it. Now, ONC could be signaling that the government agency is moving beyond simply encouraging EHR vendors to implement interoperability to actually giving them a shove into doing it.

ONC's stated objective is "The Interoperability Standards Advisory (ISA) process represents the model by which the Office of the National Coordinator for Health Information Technology (ONC) will coordinate the identification, assessment, and determination of 'recognized' interoperability standards and implementation specifications for industry use to fulfill specific clinical health IT interoperability needs."

Interoperability will deliver higher quality patient care by helping break up the logjams of entrenched profits, politics and policy. Again, ONC is coming to our rescue with the 2021 U. S. Core Data for Interoperability (USCDI), a standardized set of health data classes and constituent data elements for nationwide, interoperable health information exchange. While tagged as "United States," a close examination makes it quite apparent the USCDI can be applied and implemented universally. USCDI defined it this way:

- A standardized set of health data classes and constituent data elements for nationwide, interoperable health information exchange;

- Data Classes: an aggregation of various data elements by a common theme or use case; and

- Data Elements: the most granular level at which a piece of data is represented in the USCDI for exchange.

From an RHIT perspective, interoperability is critical for building apps that are patient-facing and can directly impact care; in this, both patient and physician benefit. Any EHR vendors which have not been focused on interoperability will find the new USCDI guidelines help define their journey toward its implementation and integration. It is high time this occurred. Clinicians have worked with the EMR/EHR technology for over fifty years, but digital technology has changed the essential aspects of medicine. We all must change; we must deploy 21st-century revolutionary technology that reflects more accurately the data and information gathered from both our patients and our processes, which will result in more precise and useful diagnoses and treatments by physicians.

HL7 has brought healthcare data-exchange standards a long way. The FHIR (Fast Healthcare Interoperability Resources) Specification builds upon and advances data exchange by adding a fourth-generation, modular programming environment and adding the information layer on top of it. This is what RHIT is intended for.

Moreover, the application programming interface, or API, greatly facilitates interoperability. FHIR's ability to isolate and describe data elements frees the data from the monolithic and often unmanageable clinical database. Using the API as the front end to access the data, innovative developers can create stand-alone applications that utilize FHIR-enabled *data elements* to deliver *information* to patients and clinicians alike, independent of the EMR.

Interoperability connects health technologies. If healthcare is to right itself and move successfully into the future, interoperability must be our destination. It is the conduit through which data and information must flow, and our conduit today is broken, fragmented, and dysfunctional. To quote Sir Winston Churchill, "Success is not final, failure is not fatal, it is the courage to continue that counts." A number of healthcare institutions are attempting to build interoperability into their operations already. Most are willing and eager to share their success with others, for enhanced interoperability benefits the entire healthcare industry. Here are a few possible solutions, all of which require everyone's buy-in.

Data ownership. After a sound legal review of your institution's policies and addressing any pertinent legal or regulatory concerns, proclaim that patient data should not be owned by any person or entity except the patient. The physician or healthcare institution can be appointed the data custodian, similar to the patient consent form, which allows the healthcare provider rights to the patient information for the term of the care.

EHR dissemination. Does Microsoft own the content you are creating in Word, Excel, or PowerPoint? The answer is no, yet some EHRs claim ownership of the data they process. Can you think of any other instance in which a software developer owns the data or information you have created? Imagine the implications in terms of data ownership if, every time one of your clinical staff accessed an EHR, there was a usage permission or a royalty fee. The issue of EHR ownership is not a new one, nor has it ever been resolved.

But it must be, in favor of the patient owning their own medical data or information, and not in a proprietary data format.

Interoperability ownership. A line from the Firesign Theatre comedy troupe went, "Which way's Goshen?" to which the reply was, "Ya can't get there from here." Think of software vendors, physicians' offices, hospitals, clinics, and so forth that cannot share information or EHR data as property owners. The governmental agency wants to encourage the building of a new roadway that will cross, and thus interconnect, all these properties, so an easement must be approved in order to do so. Consider implementing a data easement, similar to a utility easement, which requires all parties' rights and properties be respected and complied with. A utility easement, for example for internet communications, pertains only to the means of transmission, not the communications that pass through it. Any party that does not comply with the easement can be fined or forbidden access. Another means of enforcing compliance would be to create a public/private partnership with the power to regulate the data, subject to state or federal oversight.

The workaround. If interoperability is seen as an insurmountable obstacle, consider what the HIT people term a workaround. As its name implies, it is a different route to your destination. A common workaround is the application programming interface, or API. (If your software vendor is unable to provide it, your HIT programmers can do so.) The Fast Healthcare Interoperability Resources (FHIR) API standard is specifically designed for data exchange with EHRs. Because it is open-source, it obviates many of the compatibility and integration issues that beset interoperability. FHIR holds the possibility of achieving interoperability and will be discussed in much greater detail in my next book.

Policies. Matters regarding data and information integrity and dissemination must be written into your organization's policies. In many instances, policy, such as data ownership (mentioned above), whether through your own institution's governance or statutory compliance, can clarify who holds the intellectual property rights. Well-executed policy planning can also be used to require vendor conformance and facilitate interoperability. However, it may become necessary to resort to invoking policy.

Security. An aspect of safety, security for practically any reason or purpose can be invoked when patient rights are at risk. Be bold in making assertions, whether from or against any entity or situation that threatens security. A case can be made that interoperability provides the highest level of patient data/information security—for example, by producing evidence that fax machines can be, and have been, hacked, or even when the fax is sent to the wrong phone number.

Rights. Clinicians have rights. Patients have rights. Even vendors have rights, but all must be in legal and ethical agreement on the healthcare process. The clinician must never be put in a compromising position by any other parties.

Ask for help. Recognizing the ailments and out-of-date practices at their institutions, some have begun making changes in senior management and the C-suite, appointing progressive, innovative clinicians with titles such as Chief Data Officer, Chief Quality Officer, Chief Innovation Officer, and so forth. These are individuals with whom you want to work for these changes. You have a role to play, and it is unlikely you will wish to emulate Dr. Herbert Bock, Chief of Medicine in the 1971 film *The Hospital*, who cries out, "We have established the most enormous medical . . . entity ever conceived, and people are sicker than ever. We cure nothing! We heal nothing!"

Eights Steps to Transformation

We discuss outcomes frequently in this book. There are many types of outcomes, to be sure. If you undertake the changes, change management approach, and revolutionary tactics and strategies described here—in particular these agents of profound change in Part IV—you will be a driver of transformational outcomes.

Today's healthcare business model is antiquated and it just is not working well. If you do not change, your practice or your institution is going to go bankrupt, close its doors, or be forced to turn away patients. We have to get moving and change our processes, fast. In particular because of the pandemic, everything around us is changing and moving fast, fast, fast.

As Bob Dylan sang, get out of the way if you can't lend a hand.

Here are eight assessment steps you can take to analyze the health of your healthcare institution.

1. What areas are critical to the mission, and which are not? Prioritize the critical areas by assigning numbers to them— one, two, three, etc. (This should be a short list.)

2. Determine efficacy of the four tenets of the Hippocratic Code for each, and once again prioritize them.

3. Are all worthwhile candidates for change? List reasons why and why not. Be ruthless and honest; if something needs to go, let it go. Prioritize them from most to least urgent.

4. For each of your change candidates, assess their strengths and weaknesses (for all three will have both).

5. Choose the most difficult or challenging and develop a master change management plan with specific, written goals to restore the service to a five-star rating (even if it is just yours or your skunk works').

6. Recognize possible obstacles and plan for them. Identify team or skunk works members to whom you can delegate management responsibilities for the project. Assure you have top-management support to whom you can reach out for backup.

7. Undertake one at a time, especially at first. Figure out a work-flow strategy and tactics for success.

8. Have fun. You are a superhero, transforming healthcare and changing the world.

The RHIT Interview: Don Rucker, MD, Former National Coordinator at the Office of the National Coordinator for Health Information Technology (ONC), Arlington, Virginia

1. What was the most significant event or factor that determined your pursuing a career in healthcare?

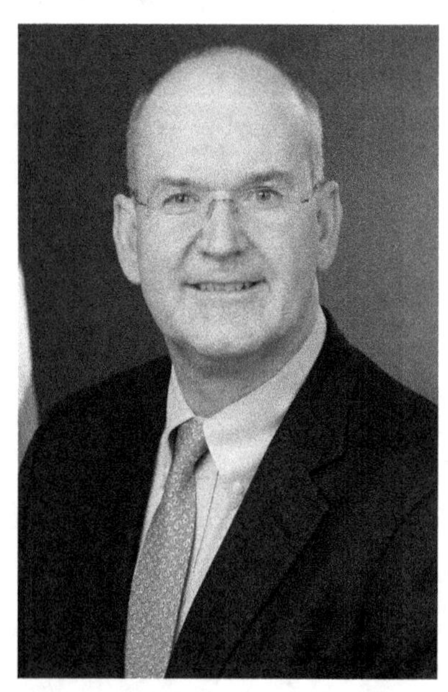

When I got to med school, what struck me as soon as I got on the ward was, wow, what these people are doing is extraordinarily labor-intensive, and extraordinarily inefficient. This was 1977, so healthcare was nowhere near as screwed up as it is today—after decades of perverse incentives and not being clearly goal-directed for the patient. There's been a lot of activity and not a lot of outcome.

I went through med school at the University of Pennsylvania for three years and the University of California at San Diego for my residency. As a resident, I knew there was something wrong and thought the answer was clinical decision support. I realized what was missing; no data to make decisions. The field was being driven by a near total lack of data. Operational data. We were using the threadbare nature of clinical trials as a way to take care of complex patients. We needed data, and it needed to be data at scale. It was not enough to have a clinical trial. It had to be instrumented data derived from computers.

That was very frankly—I'll use the word—disturbing. Clearly the skills you needed to get data were in computer software. I wanted to be part of this solution, but I was a late twenty-something doing a residency with good science skills, but no programming skills (which of course back then was extraordinarily rare). So I had to decide; did I want to actually learn how to handle data and program computers? Which is what I thought then, and still believe, is sort of a clinical informatics core skill. I decided to bite the bullet, make that career investment, and learn computer science. I was still interested in the economics, so I was very fortunate to enroll in Stanford's medical computer science program, which was just starting, and weave that in with an MBA.

2. After the pandemic is brought under control, what changes do you expect to see appearing in healthcare?

I think/hope there's ongoing movement in automation. The API work we've done under the Cures Act will be a huge facilitator. The COVID part of it specifically points out the need for rich APIs for the provisioning of clinical care. But it's not enough to just shuffle updated versions of the paper chart back and forth. What we need is a whole set of APIs to embed healthcare across geography, over the phone, and over the internet.

Understand it is not a telehealth visit in a self-contained sense, but it is informed by electronic knowledge of the prior care. Once the event has occurred, that information goes back into the patient's record, into the health information exchange and then downstream, which is also operationalized. So it's not just e-prescribing, it's all other things like labs, orders, all of that. Once you have flow of the basic information streams, you can decide what the fundamental caregiving model is.

Our fundamental caregiving model has historically been brick-and-mortar, facilitated by a medical record. But with telehealth, we can think more about population health surrounds, virtualization of population health and large parts of chronic disease care. So post-

COVID will be a lot of realization about the richness of APIs, which all technically exist but just haven't really been built out for a variety of reasons, including information blocking and entrenched business interests. It will be seen as a sentinel event for that transition, resetting the balance between virtual and brick-and-mortar models.

3. What do you think are the most significant problems facing professionals working in healthcare?

Again, I would just say we've done very little in actual automation. If you were an intern or resident in 1984, you had to read the results of every single patient, the hospital's, every single culture result, every urine test, every blood culture, every Swan tip, because they weren't alphabetized. I think we have a lot of stuff that's not instrumented in healthcare that should be when you look at the incredibly labor-intensive nature of nursing units. You know, on some level, that labor-intensiveness is almost good, frankly, in a world where we have sensors and smart beds. But the unit clerk should not be the coordinator of care in a modern nursing unit. I wrote that the single largest set of phone calls were very short patient requests. That can all be automated.

Healthcare is still way below top of license in the modern computable, but not computerized, world. Part of that, of course, is that EHRs are designed for payments and have been a sorry tool for documentation, not for automation, right?

Every other industry uses computers and networks to automate. In healthcare, their first and foremost design criteria has been documentation. It is changing slowly, but the reality is we're still paying for a large chunk of E/M code-based care. I wouldn't say people [clinicians] love their EHR, but they're deeply invested in it, which means they're anchored to it.

If you just look at labor costs in a hospital, that's where the major costs lie. Not to be cosmically trite, but the "internet of things" is coming to automation, right? So what's the temperature of the patient? What's the position of the patient? What's the movement of the patient? What's the movement of fluid in the IV? All of those things could be automated these days.

4. What are the top three reasons you continue to work in healthcare, and how might that change in the next two, five, or ten years?

Well, there are age-related considerations. But you know I have been an extraordinary optimist about what computers can do in healthcare, so I've been somewhat shocked. It's taken way too long. I thought the EMR was going to be a done deal by 1991. I guess that tells you something about my predictive powers, or the lack thereof. But we're really early on in the fundamental opportunities we ought to be implementing in order to better care for patients with computers, and more importantly, to reengineer the healthcare system so the costs are way less. The American public needs a decent deal on healthcare. So the two things that drive me are having the American public get a decent deal on healthcare, and facilitating computers.

Obviously it's been an extraordinary opportunity for me to lead the Office of the National Coordinator for Health Information Technology (ONC) with the 21st Century Cures Act, essentially mandating the rulemaking to make both of those things happen. I feel very, very privileged that the two things I've always wanted to do have been enabled in law by Congress—and that I was able to be part of the process of moving them along.

The problem is not solved. We have vast opportunities to automate, to rethink care. I think computerization software gives us lots of opportunities to be clever about the provisioning of care, injecting competition back into healthcare. And solving what we haven't solved or fixed in seventy-eight years of poor public policy.

5. How would you suggest improving and reforming healthcare?

I think you can look at healthcare reform either micro-economically or from an information theory point of view. Interestingly, either way the answer is actually the same, which is somewhat gratifying. The most efficient way is through market prices. This is known from classic microeconomics in the early 1800s. The efficient frontier, which we are not at in healthcare. It's when the consumer's marginal utility is equal to the producer's marginal costs. That's Econ 101, a market price equals marginal cost equals marginal utility from an information theory point of view.

So we have to get back to markets to solve the moral issue. The equity issue that should be uncoupled from the efficiency issues. What we have done in healthcare is mix them up, in a hellaciously bad way. We need to do what we've done in food, which is at least as important as health, right? You need food as much as you need health. We don't have a food quality program; we the public go to grocery stores and buy whatever they want at blisteringly competitive prices. Services that have a margin of around 1 percent. So stunningly efficient at handling equity with food stamps. We need that same uncoupling of efficiency and equity in healthcare. Let the healthcare system allocate resources at market prices.

Then all of a sudden, magically, we solve things like preventative medicine, the overuse of marginal technology like a hundred-thousand-dollar chemotherapeutic agent that gives you one more week of vomiting. Years on a ventilator, comatose patients, all the horrific, anti-human abuses of the healthcare system that want a market economy to go away. Nobody in their right mind would ever pay for this. You can motivate out of this purely with microeconomics or information theory, or any combination of both. And that's what we need to do.

Chapter 15

RHIT and Quality

"Good enough? Is that the standard?" asks Dr. John Thackery in *The Knick,* a Cinemax television series. The practice of medicine is not about what you're used to. It's about what makes you uncomfortable. In the practice of medicine, no two days are ever alike. Never.

For the clinician, at the end of the day the purpose of health-care is to enhance the quality of care she delivers to improve and sustain life for patients. But quality for one person is not for another. No two patients are the same, nor can they each be treated the same. Quality of care is delivered by the physician and determined by the patient.

What about quality for provider or payer organizations, or even governmental entities? Then there is the patient's viewpoint; she determines quality using implicit and highly personal criteria: Was she suffering pain from a wound infection? Did she have to wait too long for treatment? How was the doctor's bedside manner?

And there is the organizational point of view: they use widely shared performance indicators and metrics to determine quality of care. Their sample size may be as large as thousands or even millions, while the patient sample size is only n = 1. There ought to be a normalization between the two perceptions; without it, we cannot achieve truly high quality of care. Full stop.

Our task, then, is to follow this guidance, paraphrased from the baseball movie *Field of Dreams* (my favorite sport) and applied to ourselves, each of our domestic healthcare systems, and our worldwide industry: "If we build the best quality we can into it, they will come." If we raise our standard of quality sufficiently, both personal and institutional, with the intent of becoming the world leader, think what it would mean when we use the word *quality*.

Bedside Consult: The Trials and Tribulations of the Director of the National Institutes of Health

Francis Collins is, at this writing, seventy-one years old, but only in body, not in mind. As director of the National Institutes of Health (NIH), a $42 billion biomedical research agency, he presides over anything and everything concerned with the health and well-being of the entire American populace. Anthony Fauci reports to him. In his free time, he rides his Harley, often with his geneticist wife, Diane Baker, seated behind him, and plays guitar in The Affordable Rock 'n' Roll Act band.

Collins expresses concerns over the schisms that, for lack of a better term, plague healthcare. He learned in May 2020, in the depths of the first wave of COVID-19, that only about half of all Americans would take a vaccine.

The *Guardian* in October 2020 stated that among the most widely believed COVID conspiracies is that the death rate of the virus, which, according to the Johns Hopkins University tracker has so far killed millions of people worldwide, has been "deliberately and greatly exaggerated." Nearly 60 percent of respondents in Nigeria said this was definitely or probably true, along with more than 40 percent in Greece, South Africa, Poland, and Mexico. About 38 percent of Americans, 36 percent of Hungarians, 30 percent of Italians, and 28 percent of Germans felt the same.

Dr. Bruce Miller, writing in the November 2020 issue of the *JAMA*, said of the U.S. response: "Low science literacy contributes to denial of science. The relationship between anti-science viewpoints and low science literacy underscores new findings regarding the brain mechanisms that form and maintain false beliefs." While it may seem hard to accept that there are Americans who would flaunt science at their own risk, it is true. What is also true is the American spirit, captured so well in the New Hampshire credo: "Live Free or Die."

What Is Quality?

It is a word we use practically every day, but what do we mean when we say it? Has it fallen victim to semantic satiation, bandied about and used without real discernment? Let us see if we can agree on some of its tenets and get its meaning back on track. Because quality in healthcare is not like quality in any other use of the word. For clinicians, quality is protecting, improving, and saving lives. If it were applied in this most elemental way to, say, breakfast cereals, they would not be loaded with sugar. Applied to cigarettes, there would be none. Applied to the auto industry, there would at least be fewer deaths caused by faulty parts or software. You get the point.

For our purposes, there are two types of quality: everyday and revolutionary. Everyday quality, as expressed by the National Academy of Sciences, states these six objectives:

"Quality health care is care that is safe, effective, patient-centered, timely, efficient, and equitable."

Good enough, so far as it goes. No one will disagree. But is it possible for a clinician to tick off these six objectives after treating a patient? Will the physicians rate themselves, or submit to a patient satisfaction survey? What if they do not get a perfect score; what happens in a follow-up visit or when treating the next patient? Would the quality ratings even come up on a performance review? (For example, "Well, I only got a 7 on equitable, so I'll have to try harder next time.")

The point of this somewhat absurd example is to show that while performance metrics and statistics certainly serve a purpose, they do not directly impact the delivery of revolutionary care. As the poet-philosopher Johann Wolfgang von Goethe wrote:

Knowing is not enough; we must apply.

Willing is not enough; we must do.

As good as that sounds, "willing and able" is what we must do rigorously, every day. No one can be overlooked or set aside. We must perform and complete the event at hand. Revolutionary is what lies beyond what we have just concluded doing. Our quality of care must extend beyond the patient to embrace our institution: to improve our processes, which we have discussed again and again in these pages. By lifting our quality standards ever higher, and by providing quality of care that exceeds those standards with every patient encounter, we build an organization and ultimately a health-care industry that is second to none.

What is an appropriate quality standard? The primary clinical standard must shift from cost containment to quality. Higher quality will result in treatment of more people and greater access. Raising quality is elusive, if not impossible, to achieve without examining existing processes and rewriting those that are ineffectual. Changing processes makes it possible to concentrate on developing revolutionary standards; the definitions and referential touchpoints for clinical assessment and treatment are new, fresh, and challenging.

They give clinicians new viewpoints on processes and workflows, new perspectives on how things have been done, and insights into how they can be improved upon.

EHRs represent a simple yet critical example. There is no enforceable healthcare IT oversight that vendors cannot get around, which means no standards, only clever distinctions determined by the individual software vendors to assure their product's hegemony. This becomes a do-it-yourself project for your skunk works. If you worked together with your administrators and IT leaders to set new, revolutionary, strategic quality guidelines, after ensuring they are in conformance with standards bodies, government agencies, payers, and so forth, you could be in a position to demand that EHR vendors conform their products to your standard, not theirs, ensuring an enhanced possibility of platform interoperability.

Clearly, it is time we "users" begin telling software vendors to provide products in configurations we want, as opposed to what is simply convenient and conventional (not to mention profitable) for them. Needless to say, this is revolutionary, a tall task, and will take time to design and implement. It did not get like this in a day or even a decade, and will likely take at least ten years to turn it around. But it will be time well spent to raise the level of quality and safety and to achieve high-performance processes and related workflows. "Good enough" is no longer acceptable.

When Is a Baseline Not a Baseline?

Clinicians, and especially medical researchers, love their baselines in the same way elementary schoolteachers love animated GIF teaching aids. Why would they not?

A medical baseline has been defined as a data-collection process to ascertain a person's physical, mental, and emotional health. Once the initial patient data has been plotted, the clinician can refer to it at any point moving forward to determine if the patient's health in various instances has changed, and how to apply various healthcare interventions, ranging from advice to testing to diagnosis to treatment with drugs or other methods.

While somewhat useful, the major issue with the baseline is that it is predetermined at a fixed point in time. If the patient ages, say from twenty-five to fifty-five, the baseline does not reflect the changes—because if it did so, it would not be a baseline. Only the physician can interpret changes, such as weight gain or loss, the death of a spouse, the patient's increased blood pressure, medications, or because she drank four cups of coffee prior to the examination. Even more serious downsides result from the patient's relocating from, say, Brooklyn, New York, to Queenstown, New Zealand, or in some other circumstances replacing a primary care physician.

Baselines are, as pointed out, relatively static, a pre-information-age methodology that also work best with a relatively static patient. The common analogy for a medical baseline is from baseball's ninety-foot line between bases. But we are now in the throes of the data-driven age of technology and there are better ways to assess and use collected patient data. A model much more suited to our modern healthcare methodologies and practices is the Kondratieff wave.

Kondratieff waves are time-cycles that pulse in intensity, some repeating, some not, but all causing various long-, medium-, and short-term effects. Developed in the early twentieth century to chart the movement of money and investments, they apply equally well to the individual human being: waves demonstrate change. Humans, and every action we humans undertake, cause change upon change, cause and effect. Magnetism affects gravity. Stress affects cancer. Ontogeny recapitulates phylogeny, and in some Kondratieff waves, phylogeny even recapitulates ontogeny.

It is theorized that once a problem emerges as something to solve, the Kondratieff waves (with respect to a cause or need as perceived by a human) create or stimulate innovation (the effect, or means of effecting a solution), followed by the resulting technological advancements that perform the solution. These waves recur and reverberate again and again over time, creating oceanic changes, from gently rolling surf to a tsunami. Without them, we would have no advancements in medicine; surgeons would still finish an autopsy on a dead body and go into surgery without washing their hands.

Leo A. Nefiodow, author of *The Sixth Kondratieff: A New Long Wave in the Global Economy*, writes that civilization is in the sixth Kondratieff wave, which he maintains is primarily concerned with healthcare. He writes that it is "the most important engine for economic and social development at the beginning of the 21st century," and mentions its impact on Germany and the U.S. The effects of Kondratieff waves in human development and healthcare remains a subject open to new, innovative revolutionary medical research. "The leading role of health care is also evident through the fact that people in all developed countries are willing to do more for their health and to spend more money on it; and this trend will continue to grow as people will get older and will need medical care for much longer."

Strategic Quality of Care

It seems reasonable to conclude that healthcare quality is inconsistent and often amorphous. As I mentioned at the outset of this book, it seems unreasonable that a patient in Boston receives higher-quality care than one in a rural locale or small town. It goes without saying: with our existing technological infrastructure, this could be vastly improved.

What if you, as a clinician, gave the very best quality care to a COVID-19 patient but they died anyway? I believe the problem is in trying to define quality. It cannot be defined with five or six adjectives. Neither can quality be parsed; there is only one level of quality we strive for.

Quality is the strategy with which we collect, interpret, analyze, design, and deliver the best medicine possible. That is not a definition, because definitions are static and become constraints. Strategic quality is a belief, an attitude, a feeling, and the successful consummation of a healthcare process. No two of these processes are alike, so strategic quality cannot be easily defined or measured. I think we already know this. What is lacking is human initiative and a great deal of systemic change. That change is not doing today what we did yesterday, but rather focusing on revolutionizing quality, which accrues all the way up and down the healthcare value chain.

How could we not want that?

The point is, truly improving patient quality of care is contingent upon every process in the workflow. Tasks that are accomplished more efficiently facilitate other forms of improvement. Thus, for example, efficiency shortens wait time, reduces costs, and improves patient satisfaction. This creates the outcome, which we recognize with our minds, our senses, and our intuitive capability.

Yes, strategic quality is based on standards, but without knowing the definitions and points of reference for a quality standard, raising quality is difficult if not impossible to achieve. Standards can be taught, learned, and adhered to; quality should be the end result, but not solely evaluated by standards. To paraphrase Paul Simon's song, "One man's floor is another man's ceiling."

But, you say, we must have some way to determine if we are producing quality outcomes. Yes, it is important, but the old baseline way is outdated. There is a better way.

Evidence-Based Healthcare

Instead of the episodic care model, which almost certainly limits care and diagnosis and treatment, evidence-based continuity of care (EBC) utilizes a circular, rotational model that creates an endless loop of repetition to assure quality has taken place. It allows the clinician to continually assess progress, but also to make adjustments and changes in the process at any point, then loop back to assess the adjustments as well. One model, called the Deming cycle, posits a closed-loop circular system of Plan, Do, Check, and Act (PDCA). The Deming cycle is remarkable for its compatibility with the Kondratieff wave theory.

EBC delivers quality healthcare based on facts, not necessarily on inferences. It is a more modern approach to healthcare because it can gather, process, and extrapolate from data, which is the fundament of all scientific and medical practice. Intuitive care, based solely upon clinical training, is static; EBC captures data in a cumulative manner, which is always dynamic. From these chapters in Part IV and for the two chapters that constitute Part V, I will advocate for moving processes, as well as workflows, from static to dynamic, which is the way we must navigate our industry out of its past and into its future. It will be an uncomfortable journey at times, but it will be exciting to be part of moving from "good enough" to "the number one."

The RHIT Interview: Aziz Sheikh, OBE, BSc, MBBS, MSc, MD, FRCGP, FRCP, FRCPE, FRSE, FFPH, FMedSci, FACMI, FFCI, Professor of Primary Care Research & Development and Director and Dean of Data of the University of Edinburgh's Usher Institute, Edinburgh, Scotland, UK

1. What was the most significant event or factor that determined your pursuing a career in healthcare?

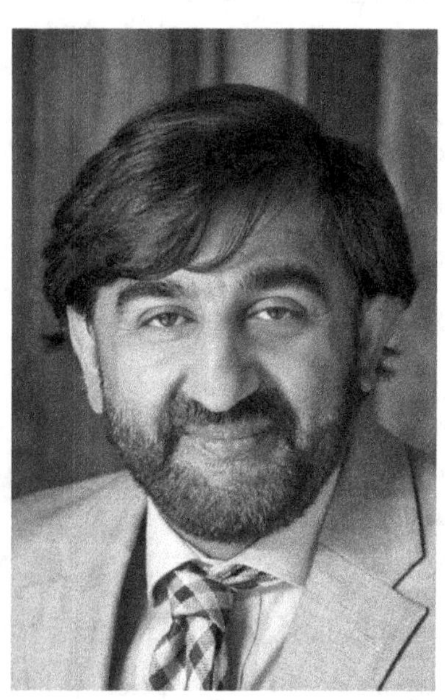

There wasn't anything particularly. Coming from a South Asian family background, medicine is regarded as a kind of pinnacle. It was what my parents wanted me to do, and I cheerily complied because I didn't have any other particular inclinations at the time. We go to university to study medicine at a pretty young age in the UK—most people are eighteen when they start. I followed my parents' advice and was very grateful for it. It was very helpful because it's really a fulfilling career in so many ways, but there wasn't any sort of "Eureka" moment.

2. After the pandemic is brought under control, what changes do you expect to see appearing in healthcare?

I think there are going to be a number of changes. Everywhere you're going to see much more use of remote models of care. That's a door I've been banging on, as have others, over the past two decades. In the COVID-19 context, it has clearly catalyzed this development beyond anybody's imagination. The pendulum will surely swing backwards, but we will be using telephones, email, and other platforms. I expect to see more continuous monitoring of our patients with long-term conditions rather than the episodic models of care that we use at the moment. I think we'll find differences in the processes for outpatient clinics, ambulatory care, GP surgeries, and PCPs. We cannot return to an approach in which we have all these people who are unwell—potentially with contagious illnesses—sitting together in waiting rooms.

I think there will be much greater use of data to guide all aspects of decision-making. This shortcoming has been highlighted in the UK. We were ill prepared for COVID-19. I hope there'll be more prominence given to public and population health.

Going forward, the UK will have a much tighter fiscal environment, so I can't envision uplifts in health resources. There's been an enormous injection of federal funding to fight the pandemic, but there are so many other calls on the government, such as bailing out the tourist and hospitality sectors. Brexit is a complete disaster that is unlike COVID-19. So I think we're in for fiscally constrained times over the next decade.

3. What do you think are the most significant problems facing professionals working in healthcare?

I think there are some really big issues, like the continuing erosion of professional autonomy. Coming from a primary care background, I also see that primary care physicians increasingly have to deal with social challenges and the accompanying "diseases of despair." In the past, many of these issues may have been nipped in the bud through the interventions of family members and religious institutions. We are also seeing growing social and health inequalities. It is thus not simply the pandemic that professionals in the UK are having to grapple with. The NHS is a fantastic institution, but you can only continue firefighting for so long. There is an incredible toll. Clinicians are well motivated, but are exhausted as far as I can tell.

4. What are the top three reasons you continue to work in healthcare, and how might that change in the next two, five, or ten years?

I work part-time as a clinician, substantively as an academic leading an applied healthcare grouping, edit a journal, and spend a fair amount of time with government bodies. I therefore have a portfolio career. It's an inherently fulfilling pursuit. I get to work with some absolutely wonderful colleagues across the UK and across the world. I find the work intellectually stimulating. There's no shortage of challenges we're confronted with in healthcare. In summary, it's the opportunity to undertake work that is inherently meaningful, to develop relationships that I value, and undertake work that is challenging and varied.

5. How would you suggest improving and reforming healthcare?

We need much better tools and real-time data sources to support health policy and planning. We know what the big disease areas are, what trends are like in other countries—what we need are the means of getting to address those issues, and prioritize and allocate resources to appropriately evaluate in near-real-time policy-level intervention.

On the delivery side of things, we need to see care reach further out into the community, outside of hospitals. We already have about 90 percent of care provided within the community in the UK, but the resources haven't necessarily followed. There needs to be much more emphasis on prevention, particularly for long-term conditions and multi-morbidity cases. For those living with long-term conditions, we need to capitalize on the expertise of patients who have the experience of living with the condition, and that of their informal caregivers who help them navigate the health system. We need to give them a better suite of tools, resources, and support to better manage their own condition. We need to move toward genuine patient empowerment and group models of care.

These are the kind of big things I think about. Certainly, from a UK perspective, these issues need to be addressed for the NHS to remain a viable proposition. It can't carry on the way it has, constantly requiring more resources, as I just don't think there's the financial headroom for governments to continue to pour money into it.

Chapter 16

RHIT and Access

I'd love to change the world
But I don't know what to do
So I'll leave it up to you

—Ten Years After, "I'd Love to Change the World"

Alvin Lee wrote and performed this song in 1971. He honestly felt he did not have what it took to change the world. All he could do was to write a song about it.

According to the World Bank and the WHO, the worldwide demand for healthcare workers is expected to double, growing to 80 million by 2030. While healthcare is the most information-intensive industry in the 165 countries the WHO tracks, our use of IT sadly ranks among the lowest of any industry. This has been true for decades, perhaps even longer than such matters have been kept track of.

Clinicians point at the fax machine as evidence of our being Luddites, and it is, but that old paper-gobbling device is hardly the culprit. To paraphrase Cassius in Shakespeare's *Julius Caesar*, the problem lies not in the technology, but in ourselves. We have become so inured to the way things are that we have difficulty thinking our way toward how things ought to be.

Yet prognosticators, writers, consultants, futurists, and clinicians themselves will quickly point out that healthcare needs extensive surgery. Unfortunately, it took a pandemic for us to see how badly we need to change our system in the most fundamental ways. Fortunately, we have everything we need to initiate the needed changes, which have already begun altering the world we knew and yet must still live in.

Of the four tenets, or critical success factors (CSFs), of the Hippocratic Code—quality, access, outcomes and investment—most of us tend away from a closer examination of access, focusing more on quality and outcomes for a variety of good reasons. Yet as I have pointed out previously all four are essential to our revolutionary healthcare reform. Access, however, may be the most overlooked, but not for good reasons, because it might just be the most important of the four CSFs for us to work toward reforming. I believe it is going to take great will and gumption to set access to rights.

What Is Access?

The U.S. government's Agency for Healthcare Research and Quality (AHRQ.gov) defines access as:

- Coverage: facilitates entry into the health care system. Uninsured people are less likely to receive medical care and more likely to have poor health status.

- Services: Having a usual source of care is associated with adults receiving recommended screening and prevention services.

- Timeliness: ability to provide health care when the need is recognized.

- Workforce: capable, qualified, culturally competent providers

No doubt these four elements of access are a good starting point for understanding our clinical responsibilities, and I am sure this definition comes as no surprise to you, the healthcare professional. Yet it is my contention that there is much more to access than what is superficially evident here. Consider:

- Our immediate objective in this chapter is to discuss how to achieve revolutionary healthcare access.

- Our short-term objective is to couple revolutionary quality and safety, access, and outcomes more tightly together (Chapters 15, 16, and 17).

- We are proposing a new way to think about the economics of healthcare, driven by the principle of a mutually beneficial investment responsibility, and through implementing a value-based system that facilitates interoperability (Chapter 18).

- Our long-term objective is transformational healthcare IT, achieved through this tighter coupling of revolutionary quality of care and safety, access, and outcomes through interoperability (Chapter 19).

Access is so important. I am convinced that we must take more seriously into account the social determinants of health, systematic racism, and gender bias. Our societies worldwide suffer from these shortcomings to a greater or lesser extent, and therefore so does our healthcare. I further contend that access is commonly disregarded or downplayed in importance by healthcare in favor of an emphasis on improving quality and outcomes. But it is also my opinion that access is the essential linchpin between quality and outcome. Access turns quality of care into good outcomes, whether for an individual or a community. All three are of equal importance, and when they are tightly coupled to one another, they make the much sought-after objective of interoperability all the more achievable.

Earlier in this book, we discussed access as a capacity management issue, which it is, and which provides us with the information technology tools to work on it. In this context, capacity constitutes the physical dimensions of the healthcare facility's ability to, let us say, manage patients in need of care (coverage in the AHRQ definition). But clinician access is also about the access provided to caregivers with specific expertise—oncology, dermatology, or ophthalmology, for example—in determining the patient's needs for treatment. Staffing shortages, estimated currently at fifteen million worldwide, are a growing concern in providing access as exhausted, overworked clinicians resign or retire, or staffing is reduced for budgeting reasons.

As illustrated by the changes the pandemic has wrought, patient access to broadband internet is important and must not be overlooked. Broadband permits patient access to clinicians and healthcare services: telehealth, patient education, and home monitoring. But unfortunately, digital access is not always available—for example, in rural areas.

The pandemic put extraordinary strains on access. It seems fair to emphasize again that the pandemic made us painfully aware how profoundly broken our healthcare system really is. Patients have lost dignity and a caring respect from healthcare. They have waited in lines outside hospitals, waiting for access for COVID-19 testing. Many were shunted to the ED, or left in examination rooms or on trolleys or wheelchairs in hallways while awaiting next steps, often for hours. COVID-19 also brought the fundamental disparities in healthcare access for people of color and economic disadvantage to the world's attention. Even those who had the wherewithal to go to their doctor were not doing so, for a variety of reasons. As Dr. Atul Gawande, writing in the *New Yorker*, said, COVID-19 testing in the United States is "as messed up as a pile of coat hangers." Both primary care and elective procedures have felt the impact of fewer (or no) customers. Governmental budgets, in particular in Europe, were insufficient to meet the overwhelming demand posed by COVID-19 and non-COVID patients. Lockdowns ensued, halting much economic activity, causing (as in the U.S.) bankruptcies and job losses. While Europeans will have to forego the traditional beso-beso greeting, far worse is the economic fallout from the pandemic—as great or greater than its impact on healthcare. In November 2020, the International Monetary Fund, or IMF, determined that the pandemic is causing the worst economic slump since the worldwide Great Depression of the 1930s.

There are many observers, both in and out of the profession, who feel our healthcare system cannot be fixed. They look at how healthcare has had fingers pointed at it for its shortcomings for decades. There is much hand-wringing, but like Alvin Lee, most wonder where to lay on their hands to initiate the changes. Access is perhaps the thorniest problem, but in my estimation it is the one that can produce the most revolutionary changes. We understand quality. We know how to manage outcomes. If we can change access, we will then be able to have a revolutionary impact on all four CSFs in the process.

Yesterday's access is a one-way, one-at-a-time, in-or-out door. Tomorrow's access is a revolving door through which pass both patients and caregivers on their way to encounters with each other—one to receive and the other to dispense quality care—and both, each in their own way, to experience a satisfying outcome. Our first task, then, is to take a closer look at that revolving door and what our problems with access really are.

Looking back to the early twentieth century, admittance to a hospital and a doctor's care was primarily available to the wealthy, who could afford it. The poor and otherwise disadvantaged were left to what we termed public health resources, such as they were (and often they simply were not). In Chapter 15, we mentioned the television series *The Knick*, inspired by the real Knickerbocker Hospital (1862–1979). Dr. John Thackery, a white doctor, performs surgery in the Knick hospital amphitheater, while his Black counterpart, Dr. Algernon Edwards, tends myriad ailments and injuries to people of color in the hospital cellar without charge. In today's world, this disparity in access stubbornly persists with respect to socioeconomic status and cultural norms. Imagine what it must feel like to be quarantined in your home watching as family, friends, and neighbors are dying all around you while you wait, inevitably, for your turn.

Yet frequently either Thackery, Edwards, or both, are brought up short at a revolving door by an alt-universe force with the name "economics." The availability of clinicians, equipment, and facilities inhibits access, and it is economics that determines whether they are available or not. We are not oriented toward getting the right value for the money spent from the investment.

Understanding Revolutionary Access

Perhaps we ought to move quickly to replace the revolving door with a patient-centered, digitally accessed portal to stimulate the revolution to improve access. Too often, the revolving door creates ships in the night: patient and clinician only glimpsing one another all too briefly. A portal is ubiquitous; it transcends time because it is available so long as there is an internet connection, and space because it does not matter where the patient or clinician are physically. We now have an intelligent door, or gateway, which captures data from every individual who passes through. All that data, once collected, provides an opportunity for informing interested parties with knowledge that exists only to be repurposed as wisdom, solely in the interest of advancing healthcare and the treatment of myriad others.

Yes, we have our work cut out for us, but the following revolutionary example proves how change can occur in even the stodgiest, taken-for-granted activities.

Bedside Consult: A Revolution on the Roads

As COVID-19 spread, hundreds of thousands of people working day jobs in every conceivable enterprise found themselves working from home. Gyms and fitness clubs saw up to 95 percent of their clientele stop working out. Cars were parked. Mass-transit saw ridership fall by over 75 percent, while city bike-sharing boomed by 65 to 70 percent.

Seemingly overnight, the nearly empty traffic lanes were given over to bicycles. One city after another started to resemble Amsterdam. Within a few months, cities like Paris, Milan, Mexico City, and Bogota were repaving, transforming their streets to favor bike travel. In the U.S., the Green Lane Project began helping Austin, Chicago, Memphis, Portland, San Francisco, and Washington, D.C., develop protected bike lanes. Bike travel on many New York City bridges trebled.

This was revolutionary access, the work of change agents who were looking quite a ways down the streets and roads to create a transportation transformation. Not everyone was on board, especially people who still preferred to use their autos to commute. Paris decided to make the new cycling lanes pop-up, meaning they could be reconfigured in the future to re-accommodate more auto traffic. This is sensible and also forward-looking, but it stands out as a revolution in the making, and cyclists are transforming the way people regard their bicycles—and cars.

An Appointment, Not at the Doctor's Office

Many patients do not look forward to an appointment with their doctor. It seems fair to say primary care physicians may not either, especially considering the average number of patients they care for hovers between 1,000 and 2,500. That is simply absurd, a situation severely exacerbated by the pandemic. Yet, oddly enough, the pandemic drove an access solution for both patient and physician: the rise in the implementation of telehealth.

Online telehealth. Providing medical attention for patients who remained at home was a solution waiting for an opportunity to solve a problem. That problem-solution, aside from its obvious convenience for caregiver and patient, resisted conventional wisdom: First and foremost, how do we incentivize it? So healthcare did a do-it-yourself to alleviate the crunch of patients seeking their doctor's counsel during the pandemic without having to make an in-person office visit. Telephone and online video interventions made the patient encounter simple and productive. Online follow-up visits were easily and conveniently scheduled, like an office visit, so they cost both patient and provider next to nothing. What is more, what we now refer to as telehealth is not confined to doctors; nurse practitioners and most allied health professionals use it as well, and are compensated for doing so.

Using telehealth lifts a great burden from the patient's shoulders by allowing them to connect from home—no driving, parking, waiting for their appointment. Patient costs are about the same as an in-person visit, and in some instances have been waived entirely. Healthcare professionals feel more productive and pleased with outcomes. And in a recent survey, seven out of ten patients favored telehealth over an office visit.

If access to the healthcare system is difficult—and we know it is—then clinicians find it difficult to deliver quality and safety. Nor can they be assured of a positive outcome resulting in what we now often term patient satisfaction. The patient is our customer, and in the modern expression of bedside manner, it is our job to deliver patient satisfaction if, in fact, that is a measurable phenomenon. The bottleneck is access. It is the most essential critical success factor.

We should not underestimate how poorer outcomes result from the patient attempting to navigate a system that is difficult to use. The world is a busy place and anything that hinders a simple, straightforward experience in the doctor's office needs to be reassessed. The top concern is always the patient's health outcome, but we must not overlook the patient experiencing a fulfilling, ongoing relationship with their doctor and staff as a by-product of that outcome. That is enhanced by access and cannot be overlooked. The ravages to conventional healthcare promulgated by COVID-19 present opportunities to learn, to grow into public health practices that will benefit all of us in the years ahead. Here is how the revolution in healthcare information technology is shaping up.

Telehealth and Data Access

Curiously, an article in the *Lancet* in 1879 suggested using the telephone to reduce and manage the number of doctor's office visits. Medicare has used telehealth techniques for over twenty years. It took the widespread use of the internet, home computers, and virtual meeting conferencing to make today's telehealth possible.

Online video appointments. Telehealth depends primarily on a video conference, but the phone is often a viable alternative and even simpler to use, especially for eldercare. Privacy rules have been relaxed to permit the video consultations using Zoom, Microsoft Teams, Apple FaceTime, Facebook Messenger, and others.

Email consults. Most patients are comfortable with email, but it is an outmoded way to message, known for its inability to communicate emotion (and therefore relying on emojis to do so). Most patients do not mind having to reach out to their clinicians with an email, but are often thwarted trying to navigate through the provider's portal. A clear solution is to ask patients their preferences in communicating with healthcare. Explain the benefits and disadvantages of each, then let them choose. Note that there is no clear policy on clinical reimbursement for email consultations. In any event, clinical updates should be promptly sent via text, email, or phone message to the patient. Whatever the medium, messages must be triaged so clinicians can efficiently respond to their patients' messaging.

Telehealth is an access technology with a bright future, so long as it is viewed as a first step in continued innovation. With regulatory rules relaxed, its use increased twentyfold. That is promising and should provide both real and virtual capital to keep telehealth going. As we become accustomed to using it, certainly many more diverse uses and applications for it will emerge.

Other Revolutionary Improvements to Access

Perhaps the greatest lasting impact of the pandemic is fewer people traveling to see their doctors and remaining ill and untreated as a result. Telehealth is a step in the right direction, but even in its several manifestations just mentioned, it is not enough to revolutionize access—and some of the reasons for this have nothing to do with the technology.

Revolutionary collaboration. Government and private research over the last decade has shown time and again that clinicians working in teams are more effective than lone-wolf doctors and on-call nurses. Effective teams of doctors, nurses, residents, fellows, specialists, nurse practitioners, allied health professionals, and support staff learn and grow more effectively when working within a collaborative environment. They form a micro–skunk works in which they can share day-to-day experiences with and about patients, spot problems in processes and workflows, and come up with thoughtfully considered solutions to problems, large and small, that they encounter. By periodically rotating team members into new collaborations on a rotating basis, they continue to spread and acquire fresh ideas and form more meaningful relationships with fellow clinicians.

Revolutionary sensing. Remote monitoring—what we used to term remote sensing—is obtaining data or information at a distance without physical contact. Whether the patient is at home or in the hospital, advancing our digital data collection methods improves our process. With artfully implemented artificial intelligence, it can pay huge bonuses when applied to diagnostics, situational analyses, and prescribing. We are just beginning to learn how to use these technologies, and it is going to take a while to get it right.

Remote sensing has commonly relied on satellite video imaging. Today, there is a satellite as well as a sensor for anything and everything; their application in telehealth is limited only by patient privacy issues. Yet on a purely data-collection basis, we can interact with and pool information from many systems: mobile phones, smart watches, laptops, and Alexa-like devices. Perhaps next is a "Siri" that can make the call to one's doctor for medical attention. These and a few existing technologies can be adapted to revolutionary technologies, as with our next topic.

Revolutionary dashboards. One very important technology still in early implementation is the clinical dashboard. Too often, dashboard displays today are static and less than informing. Clinicians are often fans of dashboards that permit intelligent tracking of patient health; dashboards today must be well designed for self-service, engaging, and predictive, since this is the only way they can truly impact patient care.

Revolutionary dashboards are not purchased from off-the-shelf software vendors. They must be custom-designed with the expert assistance of HIT using revolutionary visualization tools, analysis design, and information engineering methodologies. Dashboards must be adaptable and reconfigurable for a variety of users and changing collaborations such as skunk-works teams made suitable to particular tasks or requirements. Of course, they must be compatible with EHRs—clearly, that means interoperable—and must be capable of transforming data into information and information into knowledge, which is updated in real time, or near real time.

An ideal hospital or clinic configuration is an overarching command center informed by multiple dashboards, rescaled or reconfigured for mobile devices, individual offices, nursing stations, and other critical-need fixed locations. The home screen might be similar in design and functionality to the display used by Tom Cruise in the film *Minority Report* to track and apprehend murders. Access and manipulation is with a remote control.

Dashboards must be easily configured by and for each user or organization. In order to achieve this, they must be deeply embedded in the workflow in order to impact patient care. For example, the clinician can access their scheduled patients for the day, identify those who need specific tests or treatments, and prioritize the focus of each patient encounter. After seeing the patient, the dashboard can be used to schedule appropriate patient appointment follow-ups, all within the clinical workflow delivered by the EHR.

Revolutionary social media. Given the prevalence of Facebook, Instagram, Slack, Twitter, WhatsApp, and other online social media platforms where people congregate, innovative social media tools in the service of healthcare, which may not be immediately apparent, should not be overlooked. For example, it is possible to create specialized private groups of followers, within which ideas and insights can be shared in a healthy collaborative environment. Similar groups can be established on an ad-hoc basis between clinicians and patients under their care; in such a virtual environment, with or without video, many similar conditions and experiences can be shared in a healthy and confidential manner. Existing methods of these types of interactions need experimentation to determine what is most effective.

Revolutionary access demands that we change the technical, interpersonal, and economic bases to assure a truly connected, meaningful patient-physician relationship. We know healthcare is moving steadily toward our role of helping patients lead a healthier life, not simply preventing or treating symptomatic illness. In this progression, we must be growing into deeper relationships with our patients and our partners in public health. Our workflows must have infinite extensibility through the internet to create more meaningful human-to-human relationships.

Access is the linchpin making it possible for quality to manifest as outcome. Revolutionary access changes our healthcare world for the better. The more tightly integrated they are, the more important interoperability becomes, which lowers costs and improves care. This is our mantra, which we will continue chanting until the end of this book.

The RHIT Interview: Tiffani J. Bright, PhD, FACMI, Biomedical Informatics Evaluation Team Lead, Center for AI, Research, and Evaluation (CARE), IBM Watson Health

1. What was the most significant event or factor that determined your pursuing a career in healthcare?

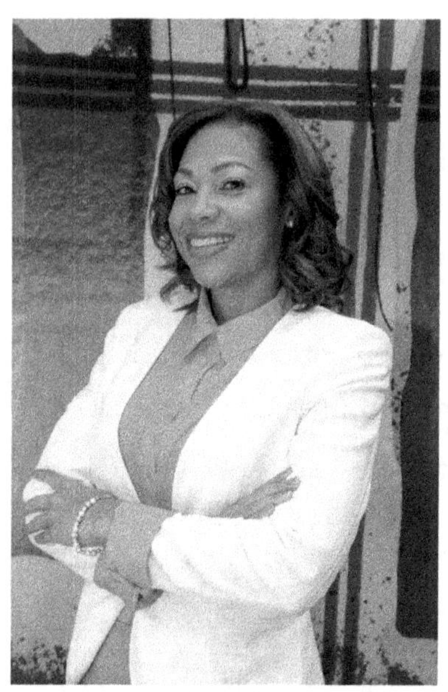

I always knew that I wanted to become a scientist; it was a childhood dream, one that my parents nurtured with chemistry sets and summer enrichment programs. In keeping with my desire to become a scientist, I started my freshman year with several science courses. As one who had always excelled in advanced placement courses, I suddenly found myself struggling with some of the material. Without the skills to fully fathom what had transpired, I internalized what was happening and assumed that I was no longer "good at science."

Fast-forward to the start of my senior year, with graduation on my mind, I wondered what I was going to do with a sociology degree. Fortunately, a family friend, who was familiar with my childhood dream, had just moved back to the area and was aware of the opening of a new school of pharmacy; she encouraged me to think about becoming a pharmacist. So, I became a pharmacy technician. Although I always had an interest in computers, using the pharmacy information system really sparked an interest in healthcare that I was unaware of and my curiosity exploded. I was notorious for asking team members about where the data were coming from; how the alert logic worked; and questioned just about everything. Becoming a pharmacy technician was one of the best decisions I made in life; it was my introduction to the field of informatics.

2. After the pandemic is brought under control, what changes do you expect to see appearing in healthcare?

We've had a lot of substantive conversations in the past few months about social justice and how racism is a public health crisis. This pandemic was tragic for all, but because racism contributes to health disparities, it has been devastating for Black and Brown communities. We can make proclamations, but what are we doing about it? Post-COVID, it's imperative that we are still committed to making lasting, meaningful changes that address how racism affects health at the systems level. For example, improving access to high-quality care, increasing preventative coverage, improving access to primary care in neighborhoods, increasing employee wellness resources, reducing food deserts, increasing pathways in medicine for Black, Indigenous, and People of Color (BIPOCs) and medical leadership positions. I think those are some changes that I'd like to see us address. Making such sustainable changes now is necessary to ensure we are better prepared to care for all of our citizens in the future.

3. What do you think are the most significant problems facing professionals working in healthcare?

Clinical documentation. I was trained to view the technology we create not as the end result but as tools that assist clinicians. When we think about the good that comes from clinical documentation, we also have to address the challenges created by the deluge of clinical documentation and how it's contributing to clinician burnout. When clinicians are burned out, there are increases for patient safety episodes, decreases in clinician empathy, and shortages in the workforce. Progress is happening with AI, but more needs to be done so that there's more meaningful insight and less noise—for our clinicians and patients.

4. What are the top three reasons you continue to work in healthcare, and how might that change in the next two, five, or ten years?

I'm not sure if I have three, but I love what I do. I entered into biomedical informatics because I was passionate about transforming healthcare. As an interdisciplinary field, informatics has allowed me to blend my knowledge, interests, and skills in unique ways to create innovative solutions. The training I received provided foundational theories and methods that I've applied to multiple problems across professional settings. In many ways a "gift that keeps giving." When I think about where I'm going next in my journey, it's continuing my workforce diversity focus, but broadening with tech + equity. I think workforce diversity and tech are critical pieces to transforming healthcare and delivering equity-centered care; that's the place where I'm headed.

5. How would you suggest improving and reforming healthcare?

The answer is very simple for me. I'd say it starts with addressing the root causes of health disparities—you know, racism. It's creating strategies to mitigate racism operating at structural, organizational/institutional, and interpersonal levels within the healthcare system. I think that's the path to transforming it.

CHAPTER 17

RHIT and Outcomes

"I'm a doctor, not a mechanic."
"I'm a doctor, not a bricklayer."
"I'm not a magician, Spock, just an old country doctor."
—Dr. Leonard McCoy, physician on the
Star Trek Enterprise

There are outcomes in most, if not all, human endeavors, whether it is baseball or quantum physics, but few beside clinicians face life-threatening outcomes day in and day out. In the *Lenox Hill* television documentary series, Dr. John Boockvar, a neurosurgeon, has operated on Chris, a sweet, gentle man, married to a devoted woman, four times for a glioblastoma tumor in his brain. Each time it has come back, and each time he has removed it once again in the hope it will be the last time and his patient will be able to resume a normal life. When the tumor appears for the fifth time in greater magnitude, Boockvar finds he must pick up the telephone and call Chris's wife to tell her it has grown back again and that the only outcome left for Chris is death. As he talks with her, his own pain of loss appears on-screen to be as profound as that of the family's.

Clinical professionals often engage in coffee-break discussions about outcomes. They are often considered the *nummus regni* of care, because they are something everyone knows and understands. We love to talk about successful procedures and their outcomes, and the gratitude of patients. Yet not all outcomes are successful in clinical terms; often they produce only partial results or cannot be evaluated using a simple measure. There are many variants in outcomes, hedged between the possibility of recovery and the certitude of death. It is left to the physician to determine what conditionals must be delineated for an outcome to be considered acceptable—much less to qualify as revolutionary. And as it should be abundantly clear by now, our goal is the delivery of revolutionary healthcare through the use of revolutionary information technology with which to transcend the everyday, to reach the greatest heights of our profession. Otherwise, outcome is just a word we use glibly, without ascribing true appreciation to its transformative consequences. We are not mechanics. We are not bricklayers. But sometimes it is possible we might be magicians.

The Outcome Misunderstanding

Leonard McCoy, that tireless twenty-third-century man of medicine on the original *Star Trek* television series, was very clear about what he was and what he was not, as his remarks attest. Yet as far back in medical history as we can have records, and clearly as far ahead as we can contemplate, there are and will likely always be great expectations placed upon healers. Many diseases, such as leukemia, were incurable until sufficient research methods found cures. Even when a particular cure had not yet been discovered, people would implore their doctors to save the life of a loved one, even when it was clearly impossible. Based on an unrealistic belief in the healer's powers and a common misunderstanding between patient and clinician, a health outcome can never be 100 percent assured.

Many doctors, especially surgeons of the nineteenth and early twentieth century, loved being regarded as superstars of medicine. Yet the patient-physician misunderstanding came about for different reasons: because of good faith and intentions. In most interventions, the outcome itself could not be faulted. Most outcomes are based upon a clinician's experience and judgment. We want to save lives, plain and simple. The decisions leading to the outcome may be the sole responsibility of the attending doctor, but might also come about from consultation and collaboration with other medical professionals and patients.

Indeed, the aforementioned Dr. Boockvar meets with several dozen neurosurgeon colleagues to view videos of Chris's brain and discuss his glioblastoma tumor. They offer comments and suggestions, but when he leaves the meeting and walks down the hall, he says to himself, "All right. Well, thank you, I think." We see, in the final analysis, that it boils down to the determinations made by the attending doctor, who is closest to the patient. Dr. Boockvar thinks back over his four years of treating Chris and comments, "We're seeing these long-term survivors . . . anyone who's living after three years with glioblastoma, you really can't predict what the cell is right now. What the tumor . . . imaging is going to look like and how it's going to behave." Clearly, there is immense room for misunderstanding of an anticipated outcome. He adds, "If I had [the time] to pause and reflect, I'd cry every time."

John Boockvar is a renaissance doctor. He is open to technological advances, but still a man who maintains a high degree of interpersonal involvement with his patients. There is utility to be obtained with new technological devices, but they are often for testing and diagnostic purposes and may not be intended for arriving at outcomes. An outcome may be what was expected or not; it may be desirable or not. But it is what it is. We practice our skills to strive for desirable outcomes, which we may or may not achieve because of the many vagaries of life. We cannot do any better than giving our work the best we have to offer in order to achieve desirable outcomes. But like Dr. Boockvar, sometimes even our very best effort, again and again, against all odds, is not good enough. The outcome is the outcome. So where does this leave us?

Experience remains the best teacher. Learning from others is, and will always be, the best education. These timeworn diagnostic tools represent only the bare foundation from which we must reach up, and out, to newer, data-driven revolutionary technologies if we are to achieve better outcomes. As clinicians, it is our charge and our objective to always produce better outcomes, and that pretty much devolves to the means and methods by which we address them.

Characteristics of Outcomes

All clinicians hope for certainty in reaching an outcome. This is possible with employing established procedures that have been taught to the clinician through education and practice—in the sense that we use tried-and-true practices. We are expected to:

- Prevent disease and injury,

- Promote and sustain health,

- Express comfort and empathy,

- Relieve the pain and suffering inflicted on patients by a variety of maladies,

- Provide care and healing for those with a malady, even if they cannot be cured,

- Strive for the avoidance of premature death, and

- Provide, if possible, for a peaceful death.

Each of these is an outcome, and assuring 100 percent excellence for each is our daily job. It is a big job, often overpowering and frustrating to the point of hopelessness, as has been the way of dealing with COVID-19. But we hope that someday, perhaps, all of our days will not be like COVID-battling days. We must reach beyond the known to assure we learn from what the pandemic taught us to make our future, and the future for those who follow us into healthcare, better. In sum, we must take what we have learned and experienced and apply it with the support of revolutionary information technology. Using revolutionary IT tools to properly deploy the EHR, personalized medicine, custom-tailored dashboards, and advanced, highly integrated systems, we will continually find new and better ways to practice medicine.

The outcomes problem. How do we know when we are delivering successful outcomes? Should we be tracking patients more or differently after discharge? Do we rank them? Is there a checklist or some other way to determine if we are getting better at our outcomes? Are we sending more patients home healthy and saving more lives? Are there diagnostic tools or apps we can use to manage our patients toward ever more successful outcomes? Is there such a thing as a revolutionary outcome? Can revolutionary HIT improve outcomes?

The solution. I assure you, all these questions can be answered in the affirmative, so long as we begin by answering the last two first.

Yes, there are revolutionary outcomes, but they differ substantially from conventionally defined outcomes. Conventional outcomes as we understand them are measurements, if you will, of performance. Numbers in spreadsheets, bar charts, graphs, analog and digital dashboard dials. Think of a horse-racing track: the winner is determined by what length the favored animal wins—sometimes by a nose. Race (or outcome) over. But consider that the animal must be coddled, walked, and cooled down until its pulse and respiration have returned to normal. Then the horse is returned to its stall for feed and a more thorough checkup by medical staff. Then it is out to pasture for some R & R.

Not very different from how we care for humans, you say? But it is. Most institutions determine outcomes on a business-costs model—for example, after a patient procedure, what is the least amount of time we can allocate them a bed? The horse, by comparison, gets the most attention and best care not only before the race but afterwards, which is what we deem the most favorable outcome of "healthcare." If the horse wins the race, it returns maximum value. But maximizing value for patients often means the institution has spent the least amount necessary to insure an outcome. That said, the amount spent does not necessarily increase the value. It is a faulty fiscal model.

There is a dirty name for this: *minimal* quality of care. There is no minimal, only maximum. We give quality of care to everything, every time. Do not let budgets and regulations alone determine patient care; the clinician has a voice in the decision.

To compound the problems raised by a fiscally determined outcome, many institutions do not accurately know what a procedure ought to cost. An apocryphal example concerns the cost of an elective surgical procedure. One hospital, creating a plan to begin offering a particular elective, reviewed what a few other hospitals said they charged. The number was around fifty thousand dollars. Word spread: this procedure returned a good profit. Then a nonprofit consulting firm conducted a survey and study of the actual numbers, which came out to just under ten thousand dollars. Charges have no relationship to actual costs or reimbursements.

Needless to say, providers rarely give pricing a thought, while patients may often determine whether or not to have a procedure based primarily on its cost to them. No business could operate without a precise, numbers-based understanding of its cost of goods sold (CGS) and profit markup. Except, that is, for healthcare. Fortunately for all, that is changing, because of the growing realization that fee-for-service has outlived its usefulness and must be supplanted by fee-for-outcome as soon as is feasible.

Going revolutionary. In order to make revolutionary changes, we must reduce or eliminate friction. The healthcare system is fraught with administrative and bureaucratic friction; it is a wonder its parts work together at all. And the greatest friction has to do with matters concerning money, because many hospitals are reluctant to operate like a genuine business. We bandy the words value and cost and profit around, but so long as there are no formal outcomes with which to measure and codify them, they remain an abstraction. Value is derived by both parties when the cost of goods sold is rendered into cost of goods paid. Costs vary wildly because it is difficult to track the number of swabs used in a day or nursing time invested in each patient. In short, there is barely any sign that healthcare demonstrates even the most fundamental aspects of a business.

Therefore, the first order of revolutionary business is fundamental, and the most difficult to adopt: we must endeavor to end episodic care, so convenient for administration and government, and replace it with the revolutionary value-based business model. Unless we get this done, there is little hope of achieving higher quality, lower patient costs, and transformational outcomes..

The four CSFs must be funded and permitted to perform at the highest level of service if we are to straighten out the problems that plague our healthcare industry. Minimal quality of care must be replaced with best practices, constantly revised for better ones. Control of the EHR data must be taken back from the for-profit software makers. It must be configurable with custom-engineered dashboards. Both must be redesigned for deep conformance with the institution's unique workflows to produce ever higher-performing outcomes. For their selfless efforts, we must champion equal pay for equal work, for all of our clinical staff who keep our public safe and well.

Bedside Consult: The Call to Care

The product and profit of healthcare human capital are both in outcomes. As often as not, one outcome can beget another, even if one is not desirable. Wartime, that most undesirable human activity, has served as an inspiration for many to rise in the call to care for their fellow beings for centuries upon centuries. In so doing, many of these brave hearts have found a need to express their wartime experiences in a variety of art forms. Two authors who volunteered as medics in times of war, both of whom chose literature for expressing their wartime experiences, were Siegfried Sassoon and E. E. Cummings.

Born into a well-to-do Jewish family, Siegfried (named after his mother's favorite operatic character), at the age of twenty-eight, joined the Royal Welch Fusiliers, an infantry battalion, as a second lieutenant. The bestiality and brutality of war quickly sickened him and drew him to write about it. His bravery as a soldier was both criticized as suicidal and praised by awards of the British Military and Victoria Crosses for his reckless feats. During a 1916 hospital convalescence, he wrote his commanding officer a letter entitled "Finished with the War: A Soldier's Declaration."

Sassoon was noted, and sometimes reprimanded, for running across a field of battle to retrieve a wounded soldier. Today, Sassoon is remembered for his blunt, forthright poetic portrayals of a World War I soldier's life, which had a profound effect on Romantic poetry and informed the modern poetry that followed, as did the writing of his fellow poet-soldier trenchmates Robert Graves (*Good-bye to All That*, 1929) and Wilfred Owen (*Poems*, 1920).

When the United States entered World War One, E. E. Cummings, an avowed pacifist, volunteered to serve as an ambulance driver in German-occupied France. A rebel from earliest childhood, when at the age of eight he began writing a poem a day, Cummings and his fellow troop were arrested by the French for what was believed to be treason, but was just a harmless prank. He was soon released. *The Enormous Room*, a novel, told the story of Cummings's captivity; it was ironic but also filled with brotherly love for his fellow soldiers. As his poetry grew in recognition and acclaim, he stated that writing poetry was a "process" not a "product." He satirically called civilization "most people," while exalting the individual and individuality.

No silver bullet. There is no quick and simple way of producing revolutionary outcomes. For the administration, a sense of participation in outcomes will pay dividends to everyone in the healthcare institution. For the clinicians, the benefits are even greater: some remain personal, while many more become success stories to share with all.

Preparing for the changes ahead. What motivates each of us in healthcare? What compels us to work so hard at keeping people healthy and alive? Clearly, there is an inner compulsion to do so, which we may or may not be able to define or convey to another. Day after day, we face the second-most fraught-upon workplaces, behind only a war zone. Perhaps that is why Dr. Boockvar seems to be making a comparison between medical personnel and military troops when he commends how his people performed in the face of COVID-19: "We all worked 24/7 to make sure that we held the line. We did not let the front fall here in New York."

Motivation could be defined as an ability to keep going in the face of adversity to achieve group or organizational goals. It seems fair to say clinicians are among the most motivated people in civilization. Healthcare workers want to do what they are doing, which is certainly not true of all occupations. Besides the well-understood factors of salary and opportunities for career development, the sense of working in partnership in a community of similarly motivated healthcare workers has a powerful impact on outcomes. Individuals feel more satisfied with a job well done when it is shared with their teammates.

In biology, this is called mutualism, when two or more organisms function in ways that support one another. This motivated clinician possesses strong feelings of purpose and value with which to inspire others to feel the same, and to communally share as if it were a form of sustenance—which, of course, it is. Mutualism promulgates symbiosis, which fosters an even deeper sense of interdependence and reciprocity. This is the ideal state for healthcare teams. It is so strong that often a clinician will forsake economic gain or greater opportunities, just to remain with their team. Which also happens to be true of soldiers in wartime.

The RHIT Interview: Karen Murphy, PhD, Chief Innovation Officer at Geisinger Health, Harrisburg, Pennsylvania

1. What was the most significant event or factor that determined your pursuing a career in healthcare?

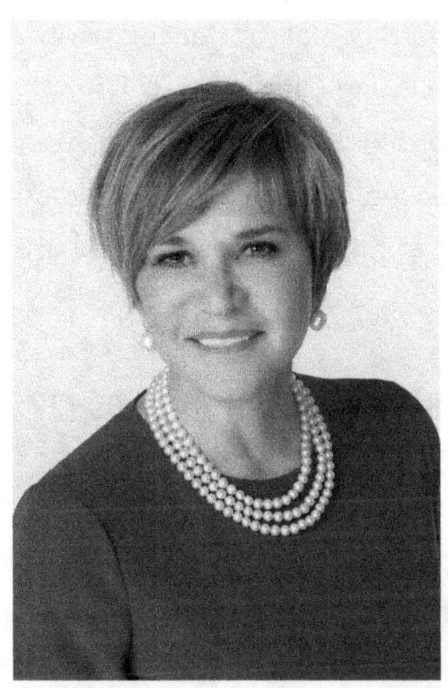

I always knew I wanted to be a nurse. When I was a freshman in high school, I worked every weekend as a nurse's aide in a nursing home. Even starting that young I realized that I loved nursing. I worked in the nursing home all through high school, and then of course went into nursing school. So I think it was just a passion for nursing and healthcare that I was fortunate enough to discover at a very young age.

2. After the pandemic is brought under control, what changes do you expect to see appearing in healthcare?

I think the pandemic has shown us, particularly in the area of innovation, great promise. I say this because we have, in the past, thought that transformation was elusive because the system was so complex. It was so difficult to change. When in reality, we stopped the entire system as we knew it within twenty-four hours. So we're going to be much more aggressive with the ability to transform, using the lessons that we've learned during the pandemic.

The pandemic has shown us that it's very important for us to wrap our arms around our patients when they're at home—in the home with remote monitoring, particularly those who are chronically ill. By intense monitoring and communication with patients at home, we truly can improve their diseased state and keep them out of the hospital. And in this way achieve better outcomes.

And finally, what we've always known but which has really never been accentuated, the fact that our reimbursement system is completely broken. I'm referring to the fee-for-service system. We did everything right during the pandemic. We physically distanced people by stopping elective surgery and by closing clinics. It was the right thing to do [for patients] and for the hospitals. However, because our reimbursement system is based on volume, it financially devastated healthcare systems. I hope we really do take these lessons and use them to change for the good.

3. What do you think are the most significant problems facing professionals working in healthcare?

First of all, workforce shortages. Second, the complexity of our care models. The way they're designed now requires us to always add more staff, which doesn't work. Obviously, there's a limit to adding staff.

So the challenge is to think digital; how do we leverage technology to help the professionals with the way they deliver care? I think the second piece that really troubles all healthcare professionals today is the administrative burden. A lot of the complexity we talk about is not because of patient care; it is caused by regulations related to patient care, and the documentation required. Some of it is for patient safety, which is necessary, but I don't think we've done a good job in controlling the administrative burden. We keep adding more to this weight, without taking anything away. So in many ways we're practicing the same way we did twenty-five years ago—twenty-five years of additional administrative burden. I think that's very, very discouraging for people.

4. What are the top three reasons you continue to work in healthcare, and how might that change in the next two, five, or ten years?

I still have a passion for healthcare and I remain convinced that we can transform it into a better place for our patients, our employees, and our communities. So I remain optimistic and, lastly, I hope to make a contribution. I've been very fortunate in my career to hold several different positions in both the public and private sector. I really feel like it's my time to give back now, so I don't see my commitment changing anytime soon.

5. How would you suggest improving and reforming healthcare?

We have the promise in digital technologies to leverage, to really create new models of care. I think that presents a great possibility for us. But the policy makers and industry leaders have to drive change both changes in the care models but also aligning the financial and the business models to meet the needs of providers by actually lowering, not increasing, the total cost of care.

We have to figure out how to lower the cost of care. It's not sustainable every year, year after year, to have increases. We must get together with policy makers and industry leaders to figure out how to get quality improvements while lowering cost. We know value is better than volume.

Part V

True Twenty-First-Century Healthcare

"Everything important in your life needs to be on a trajectory to be above the bar and headed toward excellent at an appropriate pace."

—Ray Dalio, *Principles*

It is interesting to note how much truth Ray Dalio can express in just twenty-four words. Healthcare is not on a sustainable trajectory, not just yet. The measure is different for each country around the globe, yet its evidence is undeniable. We all need to work harder toward a new twenty-first-century healthcare, because so far the only steps we have taken toward it have had to do with battling COVID-19 in 2020. Excellence remains our goal, and we must know, for ourselves, for our institution, for our patients, that we are proceeding apace. These two final chapters are intended to help you commit to making the changes that will become known as twenty-first-century healthcare.

- Chapter 18 presents the most difficult hurdle to becoming a state-of-the-art healthcare organization, one that has pulled itself into a revolutionary configuration: getting the economics fixed. Patients must no longer be considered a cost, but rather *a shared investment* with the healthcare organization. Admittedly this is not the problem for clinicians to solve, but with their help the healthcare administration can move more productively into the change management configuration to get it done and move healthcare truly into the twenty-first century.

- Chapter 19 summarizes the four tenets of the Hippocratic Code and their relationship to one another, as reflected by the revolutionary critical success factors of forward-looking healthcare. It is presented as a vision of how you and your revolutionary, adaptive, patient-centered organization can transform your healthcare delivery system.

CHAPTER 18

Healthcare Economics and Interoperability: The Bottom Line

"Before I do anything that's hard, I say: 'What's the worst thing that will happen if you do this?' And: 'What's the worst that will happen if you don't?'"

—Linda Rendle, CEO, Clorox

We have reached the point where the economics of healthcare must be forthrightly discussed. As discussed earlier in my model, the entire notion of cost is replaced with *a measurable, responsible investment by both patient and provider.* Consider:

- When the *quality standard* is based on economics, the patient experience is no longer healthcare's priority,

- When the *access standard* is rationed, it ceases to deliver quality healthcare consistently to patients,

- When achieving *successful outcomes* is not job number one, nothing else matters, and

- When we strive to assure that the patient and provider are *jointly invested* in the patient's successful outcomes and continuing good health, we are successful.

The profit motive can, and consistently does, deliver bad results. If you need an example, consider Purdue Pharma and OxyContin. Profit should never become the predominant factor in delivering patient care. I do not care to use the word cost because it is by and large retrospective. Money *invested* is more prospective. We should be looking at the spend on a patient *not as a business cost but as an investment* we are making when providing healthcare. It is not necessarily a value we, who provide and deliver healthcare, get from it. We should be thinking of the healthcare dollars we spend on a patient as an investment in that person's health. The money the patient spends is surely their share of the investment in their health. So both the patient and the healthcare organization have a mutual interest in good outcomes.

The good outcome. Here is the way it ought to work. A good outcome is not measured by quick patient turnover or low cost of services. A wellness solution may or may not end once the patient has had initial treatment. There are likely follow-ups and/or ongoing issues, so we have to think that we are continuing to partner on the patient's experience—in other words, providing ongoing care. That is our investment. If the patient did not have a good outcome, a healthy outcome, then we, the healthcare professionals, did not invest well. If we did not do the right things, the best things, the patient did not get their return on their investment. We both lose.

If you understand and agree with this investment-and-return analogy, you may already be realizing it is a bad fit with our current episodic care business model. And you would be correct. Episodic care applies a charge for a single medical transaction, not an investment in ongoing, continuous *healthcare* over time. In point of fact, that is why we call it healthcare, not medicine. To put a finer point on this transformation, we ought to be using science to promulgate *data-driven*, evidence-based healthcare.

Evidence-based healthcare, when built into a clinical work-flow, tracks and stores your procedures and their results, collects the outcomes in the system's back end, and iterates the evidence-based outcome for repurposing. If you build an evidentiary channel into the workflow represented on the dashboard, it will deliver evidence that other clinicians can utilize. Say we have a diabetic patient using a new insulin formulation. Then, using the dashboard, we start tracking it with every diabetic patient. Instead of waiting for an adverse event, we collect statistical evidence to determine the efficacy of the new formulation across the wider diabetic community, and are able to make early interventions to optimize outcomes and prevent complications.

Symptomatic medical treatment worked for many years throughout the twentieth century, but it does not work in our modern healthcare modality. It makes care cost more while it delivers less, to the detriment of both patient and provider. In order to truly serve the patient in today's healthcare environment—especially because of how the pandemic has changed so much of our mission—we need to move assertively toward a value-based care and compensation model. It will change myriad aspects of healthcare, all for the better.

One of the most important benefits from a value-based model is knowing both your fixed and variable costs. There are so many aspects of healthcare that are difficult to quantify because they are in constant flux. But knowing your costs as best you can means that now you can plan your objectives for the next two or three, perhaps even five, years. Need I mention that knowing your costs gives your organization a better idea of its economic viability?

If this is true—and we all know in our hearts that it is—why have we not already done it? I believe there are two reasons. The first reason is because we dislike change. If there is no pressure to change, we do not choose to. The second reason is because our healthcare organizations do not know what our goods and services really cost, which includes labor. Both pose monumentally disruptive agents of change.

The pricing markup. A great deal of this book addresses issues of change, and they do not need to be reiterated here. But regarding our costs of doing business, few if any truly know. Certainly not clinicians, rarely the administrative accountancy, not payers or governments. A recent study of 250 hospitals revealed that *pricing of supplies and services ranges from three to fifteen times actual cost.* For example, two hospitals' joint replacement supplies markups ranged from a high of $50,376 to a low of $16,260 for the same supplies.

It would be difficult to find any other business or industry that possesses this kind of ignorance or intentional padding of what its costs of doing business are. Yet these same institutions are unwilling to take the risk of putting a fixed price on services and guaranteeing the outcomes, fearing they cannot cover their actual costs. But what if they could better use their resources in a more consistently predictable way, by switching to a value-based care and compensation system? Most institutions know how many patients they serve; instead of collecting revenue for episodic care, they could be collecting the same or a greater amount consistently, month after month, regardless of whether the patient requires treatment or not. Imagine the increase in patients who would opt for care sooner, and be confident of the outcomes, if they knew everything would be automatically covered by their value-based coverage.

Invoicing for episodic care is expensive. It frequently involves collecting and recording vast amounts of data about goods, procedures, and labor costs to compile an invoice, which is submitted to the payer for reimbursement. Can you imagine any other business transaction with this many moving parts? Even auto accident repair bills pale in comparison.

Consider a patient having knee replacement surgery in an episodic care environment. If they ask for the cost, most often they will be told there is no way to know until after the procedure. There is concomitantly no way to know if it will be successful for some time afterwards. If the outcome is only partial or unsuccessful, the cost to repair accrues to the detriment of the patient, the provider, and the payer in both monetary cost and diminished productivity.

Compare that to a value-based system. The cost of the procedure is known in the same way a fast-food restaurant knows how much a cheeseburger with all the trimmings costs. If for any reason you are dissatisfied with your burger, a fresh one will be made for you at no cost. Value-based healthcare provides a similar warranty: for the next three or four or five years, whatever the length, if anything goes wrong with your knee it will be corrected for free, even if it means having to replace it all over again.

So why not? There is no why not. All healthcare has to do is get its processes properly assessed and defined, the accounting based on accurate data, then its workflows realigned and functioning efficiently. The great Stoic and Roman emperor Marcus Aurelius is known for having said, "The impediment to action advances action. What stands in the way becomes the way."

Some have argued that a healthcare institution successfully implementing a value-based system cannot thrive. But if we put Marcus Aurelius's perception to work, how would standing out with a different system—one that provides superior services at a flat monthly charge with an ironclad warranty—not be perceived as a competitive advantage? That would be a clearly perceived advantage.

Tracking results. Efficiencies and cost savings from a value-based system can be tracked across all four aspects of the

Hippocratic Code. A case could easily be made that value-based care delivers higher *quality* than fee-for-service. It is common practice in European and many American hospitals. For example, the International Consortium for Health Outcomes Measurement (ICHOM), based in London (with offices in Boston), is committed to value-based medicine. They say their approach "followed the development of evidence-based medicine and expanded the concept to include an explicit cost-benefit analysis, with a focus on the value delivered to patients, rather than the traditional model in which payments are made for the volume of services delivered." It is not as if it is an untested concept. It is in the works in France, Germany, Italy, Portugal, Spain, and the UK. Many hospitals profess to favor it, but still need to implement it. Certainly, it would be possible for your skunk works to design a pilot program based on my model and see how it works.

Access becomes far less of a problem when it is deployed more uniformly through the redesigned workflows: patient bottlenecks and staff shortages often disappear and work gets done efficiently. In an episodic care environment, if a treatment does not work, the patient is often reluctant to return for remediation. With value-based care, treatment becomes less about the treatment not working and the desire to remedy it. It becomes routine, not an exception; the patient steps back into a familiar workflow at just the right touchpoint, like already knowing the search term for shopping on Amazon or the correct aisle at Home Depot. The clinician wants nothing more than to resolve the problem and deliver a superior outcome. No harm, no foul.

With no-fault, return-if-it-does not-work, value-based care, the human touch between patient and clinician grows stronger. With episodic care, if the initial treatment fails, an alternative treatment may be effected. In value-driven care, we collect the data from the ineffective treatment to understand and potentially change our current practice. The patient knows which touchpoints are needed and, subsequently, the necessary care takes place. They do not need to restart at the beginning of the workflow all over again. Patient-physician trust accrues. The relationship between clinicians and patients becomes more familiar, perhaps even convivial, and you will soon find yourself consistently providing superb care. If you follow the process outlined in this book, paying close attention to the touchpoints for critical success, you revolutionize healthcare.

Superb medical care transforms into fabulous *outcomes*, which result in care that is less frequent and less urgent because it is anticipated in the patient journey and clinical workflows. To wit, it facilitates the transformation from nineteenth-century acute care to twenty-first-century health care. The value-based system assures that fixed fees fall into a predictable line. For all intents and purposes, you are delivering assured outcomes profitably.

Patients choose their healthcare institution by location (nearby) and the recommendations of others. With value-based care, it should not matter where you obtain your care; it will be close to uniform across all institutions. That is a requisite for revolutionary healthcare, and makes it imperative we assess outcomes, not cost. Superb medical care with fabulous outcomes opens the possibilities of warranties for one and all, and costs become investments.

Growth. What does "growing the business" mean? Often it means increasing revenues, year after year. Yet more often it means sacrificing one or more of the critical success factors of healthcare because it impacts goods, services, and labor. This is tired, old-fashioned thinking: hire more and buy more inventory when revenue is up, cut jobs and stock when budgets are down. The smarter thing is to closely analyze and manage the business with data and stochastic models, based on the Kondratieff waves discussed in detail in earlier chapters. Smarter, better, and less costly, while serving more patients. You can also analyze your competitive advantage similarly:

Who is your competition? Make a list of your and their perceived strengths and weaknesses, broken into functional areas, e.g., quality, physical location, services offered, and expenses, then:

- Survey your patients to learn how they decided to use your institution and what others they use and for what; is it something they could obtain from you? If so, ask why they go to the other provider. Take necessary action.

- Determine the cost for goods; how much does it cost to purchase it, stock it, track quantities, assess inventories, etc., as compared to the actual cost of the item?

- Be realistic. Some patients and their ailments are more likely to provide fair revenues than others. The variables cannot always be factored into a treatment, so accept that. Be content that you provided superior outcomes. By creating a more efficient, tightly integrated, frictionless, evidence-based, interoperable system environment, you will lower the cost of care, improve the ratio of successful outcomes, and likely amortize additional costs while expanding access to care.

Moving from the focus on budgets to the superior outcome model is arduous, but it can be accomplished incrementally. It may not be up to an individual clinician, but it is certainly a discussion the skunk works should take under advisement. What are the obstacles to creating a value-based system? Chief among them are system issues, such as software apps that demand compromises rather than facilitating best practices. Anything that would interfere with or block interoperability needs to be scrutinized. And of course anything that inhibits the delivery of the highest-quality patient care and superior outcomes.

Perhaps hospitals should share in financial risk. Patients assume risk. So do providers. When all interested parties share the risk, it coheres the value-based system. Shared risk aligns the interests of the healthcare organization and the patient. It creates value and patient satisfaction, bonding them closer to the healthcare organization. Bonding value-based care and shared risk makes practical and economic sense. The net result is an emulation of the Kaiser Permanente or Geisinger business model.

Bedside Consult: Billy Beane Had It Right

The story of *Moneyball*—the book written by Michael Lewis, made into the film written by Aaron Sorkin and starring Brad Pitt and Jonah Hill—is illustrative of our healthcare system. In 2002, the Oakland Athletics baseball team, playing on a minuscule budget, was struggling to remain competitive against teams that could afford to pay many players millions of dollars. Billy Beane, the team's general manager, meets Peter Brand, who has recently graduated college with a degree in economics. After a brief conversation, Beane decides to hire Brand to come up with a plan to turn his team's players into winners.

Beane is up against the A's player selection committee, a collection of former players and coaches whose collective acumen is the basis for hiring and firing players. Beane thinks Brand's statistical analysis of players' skills is superior to the old guys' perceptions, which are based on likes/dislikes and intuition. As Beane and Brand hire and fire players based on economic analyses—time spent getting on base instead of stolen bases, for example—Brand and Beane face incredible resistance to change from the committee.

By employing sabermetrics and developing a new strategy for who would play where, Beane, in one season, was able to turn the A's—with a miniscule annual budget of about $40 million—into a winning team, beating clubs with budgets three and even five times larger. The A's made it to the playoffs, dispelling criticism and proving that baseball was emerging from the dark ages of subjectivism into a game that could be played analytically and with saber-sharp precision. It was a move that proved it did not matter if you picked an expensive player. What mattered was recognizing that an inexpensive player, playing in a strategically identified position, could play better. Baseball was no longer about big money; it was about smarts. Against tough odds and long-held resistance, the game had changed.

Science, Not Guesswork

The *Moneyball* story points to two important conclusions for healthcare. One, experience and intuition are no longer the best or only skills for practicing clinicians. Perhaps they were fifty or a hundred years ago, but technology has begun transforming our industry. Data and statistics are fundamentally reliable and must become our decision-making platform, not opinion and personal experience. What has changed in baseball has, and is, changing healthcare as well.

Trusting the science has proven itself in baseball again and again. The Boston Red Sox used sabermetrics to win four World Series championships, while my home team, the New York Mets, have not done as well over the same period, having failed to embrace analytics. (But now, with Steve Cohen becoming owner, expect to see more hedge fund–inspired analytics brought to the team from Queens.) As recently as 2020, the Tampa Bay Rays, following the science, nearly won the World Series. Jason Gay wrote in the *Wall Street Journal*, "There's a reason the Rays rely so hard on analytics to make decisions: if done right, it requires a lot less money." Quality before profit rings true again.

Two, you must have your ducks in a row to make these kinds of changes. You *must* know what everything costs or at least how to find out. If you do not know what things cost, whether it is Q-tips or an OR nurse, you cannot build a value-based budget. Without budgeting, you do not know what your operating expenses are. You cannot determine the value of what you are spending on healthcare. You cannot amortize large-scale outlays. And if you do not know these things, you cannot know how much to fairly and accurately charge patients.

Needless to say, you do not want to learn your organization is overcharging. There is too much at stake: the administrative costs to revise the accounting, the damage to both the clinician's and the organization's reputations. You cannot just make up costs; it will catch up with you eventually, one way or another. Besides being unbusinesslike, besides being irresponsible, it is unethical and fraudulent. Clearly this is a matter for the administration and payers, who often find themselves in an adversarial relationship. But clinicians ought to take an interest in the operational aspects of their occupation as well, for all of these reasons. Personal and business reputations are on the line. Value-based accounting obviates many of these situations because everything is held to the evidence-based standard.

Tallying charges for a plethora of fixed costs for a deliverable is administratively expensive. It involves capturing vast quantities of data from multiple sources about goods, services, and labor to compile into a price, which is submitted to the payer for haggling and eventual agreement. Can you imagine any other business transaction so complex?

Value-based service puts the emphasis on the patient and outcomes, which drives profit. A case in point: a doctor in Paris determined her patient needed bypass heart surgery. The man was operated on and spent three days in the hospital, then was sent to a rehabilitation clinic. He was told he could stay in the rehab until he was confident enough of his recuperation to return home. He asked how he would know when that might be. The nurse told him—when he could safely descend the stairs from his fourth-floor apartment to the ground floor to check his mail, and go back up.

Integration

It should be clear that best practices, evidence-based treatment, and value-based care in general lend themselves better to a more efficient, productive, and less costly integrated process than episodic care. They are the essence of revolutionary healthcare, based upon a rock-solid information technology foundation. How the three are configured will certainly vary from one healthcare organization to the next; the important thing is to get your skunk works busy defining them as part of the new revolutionary HIT business plan you intend to propose, because:

- *Revolutionary quality and safety* improves your institution's game;

- *Revolutionary access* makes that integration tighter;

- *Revolutionary outcomes* help you successfully market your clinicians and your organization to the world; and

- *Revolutionary patient-provider investments* in outcomes increases respect and affiliation for your institution.

Each of these is achievable once you have tightly integrated them into your new RHIT Methodology, processes, and workflows. The tighter we can make the integration from quality to access to outcome, the sooner and better we can achieve better ROIs. Why?

Because we have reduced friction between disparate parts of the system. Interoperability facilitates less friction.

Interoperability

First, let me say I do not think not-for-profit healthcare institutions provide greater efficiencies or greater value than for-profits, or vice-versa. The issues that must be resolved for moving toward interoperability are clinical, technical, and systemic. Interoperability is in itself a technical, systemic solution to reducing organizational friction because it renders the entire enterprise transparent and thus more efficient. Putting interoperability ahead of financial objectives would genuinely improve the investment in patient health.

- Embrace change.

- Employ skunk works strategies for change.

- Hold the Hippocratic Code to the highest standards.

- Use the Chaiken RHIT Methodology as a model to analyze touchpoint strengths and weaknesses.

- Deploy your own version of the RHIT Methodology.

- Begin reducing systemic friction by creating tighter integration.

- At the optimal touchpoint, begin converting integration into interoperability.

Superb Healthcare

Some might believe there is an inherent moral hazard in practicing medicine. A doctor is often in the position to prescribe a treatment that may or may not be successful. It may cause more harm than good. It may result in the patient's death. And in some cases, the decision to perform the procedure may be based not so much on the patient but on the budget available to that healthcare facility or the payer rules that apply to a particular patient.

Of course, all are moral hazards because they ask the clinician and/or the chief medical officer to make the tough decisions. The doctor may become biased regarding the decision in favor of available resources for the procedure. That is the inherent bias in episodic care. It is bad for the doctor, it is bad for the patient, and it is bad for the healthcare institution.

Yet if the doctor were practicing in a value-based care environment, that moral hazard would be severely mitigated because she would be using evidence-based medicine to assure the correct diagnosis and data-based decision-making. The profession, collectively, may assume that some routine tests are de rigueur, without thinking if they are really needed. That becomes a moot point in an evidence-based system. Performance and feedback are also part of the medical record, as mentioned earlier in the dashboard example, so everyone concerned can see what worked and what did not.

Coding. It runs even deeper, encompassing the codes, which are designed for documenting care for reimbursement or budgeting. Even when based on ICD-10, the purpose of codes is billing: to make a compensatory determination, not a medical one. Coding is a necessary evil, so to speak, because of the need for accurate classifications, but the coding system could also be used clinically, for tracking and measuring. An expanded data-collection and classification system could utilize codes to administer the clinical assessments and build a knowledgeable repository. The information it might contain would permit comparison within a sample, or chart trends and progressions, establish comparisons to historical instances, and fairly assign financial assets. The doctor or nurse will never have to justify ordering a test or additional procedure, because the evidence will have already pointed to it.

The bottom-line issue is, we spend a lot of money. We are always asking ourselves, how can our healthcare program save money or improve profitability? We do not know how to determine if we are getting enough bang for our buck.

I ask you, why does it matter? If the evidence-based diagnosis says, "If we do these things for people, they are going to have better outcomes, a better quality of life," that is simple enough. It means when I decide to spend a few dollars to do something, I am probably creating value. My patient is getting value. My employer is getting value. Society is getting value. So the question is not how much money we *spend* on healthcare, nor if we are generating profits. The question is, *how much value do we give and get* from our investment in providing healthcare? Right? And the focus should be on optimizing value, not minimizing cost, right?

If we optimize value, we will naturally decrease costs. That is just true. There is a lot of proof. A lot. There so many things we can change. But until we begin to change them, how can we know what difference they will make?

The RHIT Interview: Priyanka Grover, MBA, Head of Analytics at SingHealth, Singapore

1. What was the most significant event or factor that determined your pursuing a career in healthcare information technology?

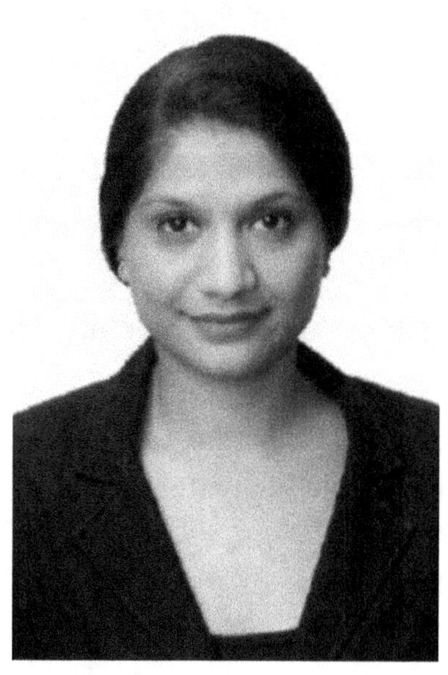

My encounter with the healthcare industry started when I joined Cerner in 2005. I was intrigued by the healthcare IT systems and had the opportunity to understand a healthcare ecosystem from a system perspective. The driving factor was the complexity of the domain, and an ocean of knowledge I had to dive into to build my expertise over a period of time.

2. After the pandemic is brought under control, what changes do you expect to see appearing in healthcare?

The pandemic has highlighted several areas that need to change, especially the importance of coordinated care. Access to the right information at the right time can improve patient outcomes tremendously. I believe patients can be empowered to manage their health better.

3. What do you think are the most significant problems facing professionals working in healthcare?

Most healthcare professionals face burnout problems. We are dealing with ever-growing demands for healthcare services, yet the manpower resources are limited. Emerging technology and innovations do hold the promise to solve some part of this issue. But the human touch is essential in this industry; we must embrace technology without losing the human-centric approach.

4. What are the top three reasons you continue to work in healthcare, and how might that change in the next two, five, or ten years?

Working in this industry has made me realize that even though we focus on IT, whatever we build is for better patient outcomes and for a greater good. The people in this industry usually have their hearts in the right place. The essence of humanity is helping each other, especially when there is pain and suffering.

I hope we will better understand the holistic well-being of individuals and move towards better health, rather than the need for healthcare itself. This will bring fundamental changes in the care models, as well as in our patients' perceptions and attitudes about their own health.

I wish to continue working in this industry and focusing on social impact and community health.

5. How would you suggest improving and reforming healthcare?

Any improvement or reform requires a catalyst. It may be radical or at a steady pace. From my perspective, we need a few radical changes where we embrace innovation and technology without losing the human touch. At the same time, we must keep trying to redefine health holistically and empower each individual to care for their own well-being. We need to embrace that the whole is greater than the sum of its parts. We must develop new models of care with this understanding.

The Connected, Adaptive Healthcare Organization

As *Star Trek: Deep Space Nine*, season five, episode sixteen, opens, a twenty-fourth-century conversation is underway aboard the Deep Space Nine space station between Captain Benjamin Sisko, Doctor Julian Bashier, and Doctor Lewis Zimmerman, a visiting technologist-physician. They are discussing a medical holographic program that can assist the ship's doctor during emergencies. Zimmerman attests to the hologram's far greater abilities; he states it can replace the human doctor. He says, "I'm surprised you don't have one on station."

Captain Sisko says, "The station facilities are Cardassian in origin. Most of our equipment is incompatible with Federation biology."

Hit pause. Does this sound familiar?

Sisko is clearly uncomfortable with the notion of a hologram for the station's medical doctor. Undaunted, Zimmerman continues, "Why is everyone so worried about holograms taking over the universe?" He is there to ask permission to install an emergency medical hologram, or EMH, which will be simulated based on the living, extraordinary physician Dr. Bashier. "It is nothing less than a shot at immortality," he chortles. Then he requisitions access to the "mainframe computer" and a "high-speed data link."

Hit pause. Then everything changes.

Or does it? Four centuries into the future, technology incompatibilities persist. The human doctor, perhaps fortunately, remains the model upon which advanced technology is based.

"The more things change, the more they stay the same," said writer Jean-Baptiste Alphonse Karr in the nineteenth century. And of course he was right. We are able to envision our future based upon what we have learned in the past and what we know in the present. This is the unique mental capability humans possess that, to the best of our knowledge, other species do not. They are not able to see the forest for the trees, but we can. But do we?

Where to begin? If you have understood the evolution of the Hippocratic Code critical success practices, you probably have noted the parallel progression: first with quality and revolutionary change; second with access and adaptation; and finally with outcomes and transformation. *Star Trek*'s Zimmerman is proposing what seems to be revolutionary change, but it is not; he simply has to shift Sisko's thinking about how things have already changed. His proposal is in fact an adaptation, in this case of a human doctor's knowledge and experience into a holographic image. Not so different from how we now think about implementing artificial intelligence.

This book is not a handbook, nor is it a stepwise guide to how to fix healthcare. There are too many variables and nuances in the way healthcare operates to make blanket pronouncements. My purpose in writing this work for you is to present a vision of how *you and your organization can transform your healthcare*. It is a reimagining of ourselves and our work. Our personal sense of worth. Our outcomes. If you have read this far, I hope you have already begun reimagining how you can make your workplace better, far better than it has ever been.

Think about how good it would make you feel if you decided to clean up your office. You put away stacks of journals, shelve new books, organize your desktop, perhaps dust and vacuum, rearrange the furniture, finally give your computer its latest upgrade. You're pleased at how much better everything looks and feels, which in turn enables you to organize and manage your workflow for higher efficiency and productivity. You are now freed from the constraints of disorganization, and your mind is popping with great new ideas and plans. In other words, straightening up your office has also refreshed your mental processes. You are ready to stir up a revolution in your work life. You have set out on the road to becoming a more adaptive knowledge worker.

Toward a Revolutionary Tomorrow

It would be something of a stretch to say we are engaged in a healthcare revolution right now, today. Yet there are clear signs of change in this direction (see this chapter's Bedside Consult), enough to give us hope in a full-scale launch into revolutionary healthcare:

- What will healthcare be like in two years? Will we still be mired in COVID-19?

- What about five years from now? Will we in healthcare still be nose to the grindstone, doing the same-old, same-old? Or will we have changed to a value-based model?

- What will those who proclaim the "new normal" see in our civilization a decade into the future? Will we, in healthcare, be able to say we conquered the virus—perhaps all viral disease—maybe even cancer? Do we have any idea what might be possible once we have working interoperability?

These are serious, not fanciful questions, which is why I asked them of the eighteen thought leaders interviewed throughout the book. They are touchpoints we clinicians and concerned citizens need to not be just thinking about, but rather using them to create the change agents necessary to make them come true.

Bedside Consult: "Only Connect"

"Only Connect." These last two words in E. M. Forster's 1910 novel, *Howards End*, have resonated with people for over a century. It sounds simple, but connecting has been unalterably changed for us since the rise of the public internet in the 1990s. We humans are biologically wired to be social creatures; our desire is to be together, and digital socialization cannot and will never replace this fundamental need. We may have more and better ways to connect with others, but the connections are all too often more complex and unfulfilling. Therefore, we need to be rigorous in selecting our communication channels, weeding out those that cannot meet our criteria for importance. This is especially critical when managing patient care workflows.

The issues healthcare workers most frequently encounter have to do with human-social connections: overworked, understaffed, no mentoring, an incompetent boss, not having enough time to attend to core responsibilities. Being overworked is likely the root cause of the problems in the other areas. We need to learn how to slow down and reflect upon what we are doing from the perspective of time, mentioned earlier. When we manage time better, we make it possible to connect better. We will manage time better when we concern ourselves with patient care, rather than invoices created by the administration.

But "only connect" has to be seriously analyzed in terms of workflow. Think of workflow as connective tissue, essential unto itself but also to what it connects: from the quality of data entering, through the EHR to the outcome. Data, at any point in the process, can be abstract and difficult to interpret, both of which must always be a consideration. That is why data alone is not the most important element; what is most important is the information it produces in order to support the repository of knowledge, which imbues the clinician with the wisdom essential in consistently making right decisions. Data must always be collected for a specific purpose, not simply because it exists, a fact that eludes many. Even information gathered in a computer cloud without context is gathered pointlessly. Knowledge can be effectively imparted in a variety of media formats, ranging from casual conversation to white papers to books and audiovisual media. All are useful, especially if they can be accessed more than once to connect with even more clinicians who have a desire or a need to know.

The pervasiveness of dashboards is a good sign, but the technology must be developed to fit clinical needs, not the other way around. Much of the purpose of using dashboards focuses on data reporting for administrative use. This does not benefit the patient or the clinician. This is why it is essential that clinical staff, perhaps as a skunk works project, design and implement their own custom dashboard, built upon a sound software foundation, to focus on collecting and sharing information and knowledge, rather than displaying unfocused data. It is highly likely that HIT would be happy to partner with clinical in designing state-of-the-art dashboards, linked across processes, that inform enterprise-wide decision-making at the individual points of care that deliver consistent, desirable outcomes.

Adaptation

An adaptive healthcare enterprise is one in which change is the norm, not the exception. If something is not working, or if it is working poorly, change it. Now. Consider the impact of not making changes when the need is clearly recognized: politicians have presented over nine hundred constitutional amendments to eliminate, or at least amend, the electoral college, yet it remains like a stubborn donkey in the middle of the road to more progressive elections.

The adaptive organization is always looking outside itself, scanning emerging health concerns (like a possible pandemic) and the socioeconomic landscape (for instance the implications of an increase in unemployment), out at least twenty years. Healthcare knows it has problems but recognizes that they can be solved with the partnership of HIT and its well-honed tools, from helping provide new software applications to analyzing data.

Adaptive evolution is recognizing and solving problems. It is a primary life force in every living plant and animal. For healthcare to achieve purposeful adaptive evolution, we must understand how things got the way they are. There were reasons: some were likely good reasons, but some were thoughtlessly or carelessly instituted. Once understood in the light of preserving what is good and getting rid of what is not, then we can take steps to intelligently improve our ailing processes. That is adaptive evolution.

However, humans sometimes get stuck in their ways and either cannot or will not take the adaptive steps. In such cases, one of two things happen: one, the entity fails to sustain life (extinction), or two, it undergoes revolution. This is as true for a flower as it is for a hospital. For our solution, we favor revolution. We are not talking about an overthrow, but something more on the order of a phoenix rising from the ashes. It comes as no surprise to any citizen of the world that healthcare is in profound need of change. What is lacking is the leadership and the strategy to do so. For this, we need a full deployment of the HIT resources: hardware, software, thoughtware. We cannot stick our collective heads in the sand if we are to thrive.

What's at Stake: A Lot

Who knows how long COVID-19 will last? Or when the next pandemic will arrive? We certainly do not know at this time, but what we do know is that you, the clinician, the administrator, the analyst, and the patient hold the future of your country, if not the entire world, in your hands. Honestly, you really do. We are going to undertake an exciting, meaningful project that, to paraphrase the Silicon Valley mantra, is going to change the world. Once we have become a revolutionary, connected, adaptive organization, the next inevitable step is to become transformational. It is the next logical step. Its evolution cannot happen any other way.

We simply cannot afford to decline the challenge. These changes will not happen overnight, nor are any of them optional, as I am certain you are already aware. But it can happen, and with your help it shall. Will you be content to bear the responsibility of doing nothing to change the healthcare environment? Or will you feel the energy and optimism that comes from knowing you have, and will continue to have, played a role in transforming healthcare?

The takeaway from reading this book should be clear to you by now: we have an incredible ability to change ourselves and our environment. As individuals, whether we work in healthcare or not, we must be change agents. Now it is time to create substantial change in the healthcare workplace. It is not too late, or if you think it is, then better late than never. We need not be disruptive. The path to meaningful change in healthcare begins with revolutionary thinking that makes it possible to enhance our connectivity, and therefore makes us more adaptable, individually and collectively, to a transformed healthcare environment.

The Greeks often used the term *phronesis*, which for them meant practical wisdom. It seems like a step up from common sense, which may refer more to an inner sensibility than an acquired wisdom. Yet both point us in the proper direction with healthcare. What is the price of not changing? Likely more of the same-old, same-old, and for sure the massive, crippling unpreparedness we experienced with the 2020 pandemic, again and again. Healthcare is the most important business in America and much of the world, and once we get it on the right track it will be a beacon to any and all individuals and enterprises.

As Captain Jean-Luc Picard so famously said, "Make it so." It is up to you.

The Center for Healthcare Information Security

Although you have come to the end of this book, it is only the beginning of your journey to a better, stronger, more efficient healthcare. As you know by now, this is not a how-to book; it is a *why-to*. If you are ready to take the next steps, I am here for you at the Center for Healthcare Information Security (CHCIS).

The CHCIS is a nonprofit 501(c)(3)organization. Our mission is to develop and promote, through education, training, and certification programs, the best practices and standards covering the fundamental principles of healthcare cybersecurity and its related disciplines necessary to protect personal health information. Cybersecurity, often overlooked, must be part of the core principles in any movement toward a new healthcare organization. It is as important as the Hippocratic Oath and Code, which is the focal point of my next book.

If you are ready to get started, our work at the Center can benefit you. Here are some ways we can work together to get your transformation underway:

We develop and promote customized courses of study and continuing education programs for healthcare professionals. These programs are predicated on healthcare cybersecurity, then progress into working with the principles and practices described in this book. Our programs are modular and incremental, structured like the five Parts of *Navigating the Code*, giving you and your organization the ability to learn at your own pace and adapt the Chaiken Methodology to your own needs and goals.

We can conduct custom research and evaluation of your organization to develop the touchpoints essential for implementing your change management program. We recommend and implement educational programs in the fundamental principles described in this book, beginning with a high-level assessment of your healthcare cybersecurity, which as you know is essential to protecting personal health information. With this requirement satisfied, a change management strategy can be designed.

Our programs include examinations for professionals who desire certification of proficiency, and a certificate of proficiency or other similar level of distinction in healthcare cybersecurity or the entire Chaiken Methodology implementation.

We will engage with you in any activities that help professionals in their work on healthcare cybersecurity, change management, and organizational transformation, using RHIT. Our goal is to lend assistance however we can in achieving your goals.

For more information, please visit the Center's website, http://chcis.org/.

Endnotes

(All active links to the endnotes can be found at https://navigatingth-ecode.com/further-reading/endnotes/. They are accurate as of May 6, 2021.)

Introduction and Preface

Henninger, Daniel, "Caught Napping by Coronavirus," Wall Street Journal, April 8, 2020, https://www.wsj.com/articles/caught-nap-ping-by-coronavirus-11586387404.

"The Computer Algorithm That Was Among the First to Detect the Coronavirus Outbreak," CBS News, April 27, 2020, https://www.cbsnews.com/news/coronavirus-outbreak-computer-algorithm-ar-tificial-intelligence.

Belk, David, "True Cost of Healthcare," accessed February 12, 2021, https://truecostofhealthcare.org/hospital_financial_analysis.

Slate, Jeff, "John Cleese on Why Open Offices Are Among History's Greatest Mistakes," *Wall Street Journal*, October 28, 2020, https://www.wsj.com/articles/john-cleese-on-why-open-offices-are-among-historys-greatest-mistakes-11603899772.

"Clarke's Three Laws," Wikipedia, accessed February 12, 2021, https://en.wikipedia.org/wiki/Clarke%27s_three_laws.

Chapter 1: The Current State of Worldwide Healthcare

Peck, M. Scott, *The Road Less Traveled: A New Psychology of Love, Traditional Values, and Spiritual Growth* (New York: Simon and Schuster, 1978).

"Belarus' Economy Can Face a Severe Shock, Says World Bank," World Bank, May 26, 2020, https://www.worldbank.org/en/news/press-release/2020/05/26/belarus-economic-update-spring-2020.

Nabil Shaaban, Ahmed, Bárbara Peleteiro, Maria Rosaria O Martins, "COVID-19: What Is Next for Portugal?" *Frontiers in Public Health*, August 21, 2020, https://doi.org/10.3389/fpubh.2020.00392.

"World Population Ageing 2019," United Nations Department of Economic and Social Affairs, 2019, https://www.un.org/en/development/desa/population/publications/pdf/ageing/WorldPopulationAgeing2019-Highlights.pdf.

"The Complexities of Physician Supply and Demand: Projections from 2018–2033," Association of American Medical Colleges, accessed February 12, 2021, https://www.aamc.org/data-reports/workforce/data/complexities-physician-supply-and-demand-projections-2018-2033.

Bureau of Economic Analysis, U.S. Department of Commerce, accessed February 12, 2021, https://www.bea.gov/.

"*The Road Less Traveled* Quotes," Goodreads Inc., accessed February 12, 2021, https://www.goodreads.com/work/quotes/2747475-the-road-less-traveled-a-new-psychology-of-love-traditional-values-a.

Chapter 2: Healthcare IT: The Digital Conundrum

Interviews with John Gantz, Senior Vice President, International Data Corporation, conducted May 5, 2020, and November 15, 2020.

Chapter 3: The Management of Change

Martin, James, *The Wired Society* (Englewood Cliffs, NJ: Prentice-Hall, 1978).

Harven, Michelle, "From Galileo to Dr. Fauci: The History of Science Denial and Conspiracies," National Public Radio, May 19, 2020, https://the1a.org/segments/from-galileo-to-dr-fauci-the-history-of-science-denial-and-conspiracies/.

"Hospital Service Line Organization: Innovation in Approaches and Strategy," Modern Healthcare Insights, 2012, accessed February 12, 2021, https://www.modernhealthcare.com/assets/pdf/CH81353810.PDF.

"*The Road Less Traveled* Quotes," Goodreads Inc., accessed February 12, 2021, https://www.goodreads.com/work/quotes/2747475-the-road-less-traveled-a-new-psychology-of-love-traditional-values-a.

Open Notes, "Open Notes," accessed February 12, 2021, https://www.opennotes.org/.

"HHS Extends Compliance Dates for Information Blocking and Health IT Certification Requirements in 21st Century Cures Act Final Rule," U.S. Department of Health and Human Services, October 29, 2020, https://www.hhs.gov/about/news/2020/10/29/hhs-extends-compliance-dates-information-blocking-health-it-certification-requirements-21st-century-cures-act-final-rule.html.

Nefiodow, Leo, "Kondratieff Cycles," accessed February 12, 2021, https://www.kondratieff.net/kondratieffcycles.

Drucker, Peter, *Managing in a Time of Great Change* (Boston: Truman Talley Books/Plume, 1998).

Dalen, James E., and Joseph Alpert, "Medical Tourists: Incoming and Outgoing," *American Journal of Medicine*, 2019; 132: 9–10.

Chapter 4: A CAT Scan of Today's Healthcare Business

Murthy, Vivek H., *Together: The Healing Power of Human Connection in a Sometimes Lonely World* (New York: Harper Collins Publishers, 2020).

Porter, Michael E., *The Competitive Advantage: Creating and Sustaining Superior Performance* (New York: Free Press, 1985).

Gabbard, Philip, *Thrivation: The Everlasting Philosophy of Providence + Privilege* (Amazon Independent Publishing, https://www.amazon.com/Thrivation-Everlasting-Philosophy-Providence-Privilege/dp/B08N9PZMSC, 2020).

Nefiodow, Leo, "Kondratieff Cycles," accessed February 12, 2021, https://www.kondratieff.net/kondratieffcycles.

"Skunk Works," Wikipedia, accessed February 12, 2021, https://en.wikipedia.org/wiki/Skunk_Works.

Dalio, Ray, *Principles: Life and Work* (New York: Simon & Schuster, 2017).

Christensen, Clayton M., *The Innovator's Dilemma: When New Technologies Cause Great Firms to Fail* (Boston: Harvard Business Review Press, 2016).

Chapter 5: Implementing Revolutionary HIT Change

"Warren Buffett Quotes," Goodreads Inc., accessed February 12, 2021, https://www.goodreads.com/quotes/47192-should-you-find-yourself-in-a-chronically-leaking-boat-energy.

"Paul Romer Quotes," Wikiquote, accessed February 12, 2021, https://en.wikiquote.org/wiki/Paul_Romer.

Chapter 6: Transforming Today's Healthcare with HIT: Systems Thinking

"Peter Drucker Quotes," Goodreads Inc., accessed February 12, 2021, https://www.goodreads.com/quotes/76788-results-are-obtained-by-exploiting-opportunities-not-by-solving-problems.

"Jay Wright Forrester," Wikipedia, accessed February 12, 2021, https://en.wikipedia.org/wiki/Jay_Wright_Forrester.

"VisiCalc of Dan Bricklin and Bob Frankston," History Computer, accessed February 12, 2021, https://history-computer.com/visicalc-of-dan-bricklin-and-bob-frankston/.

"Avedis Donabedian," Wikipedia, accessed February 12, 2021, https://en.wikipedia.org/wiki/Avedis_Donabedian.

Chapter 7: A Revolutionary Process

Follett, Ken, *The Pillars of the Earth* (New York: William Morrow, 2012).

Chapter 8: Transformational Outcomes

"*I Ching*," Wikipedia, accessed February 12, 2021, https://en.wikipedia.org/wiki/I_Ching.

Lenox Hill (TV Series), Netflix, accessed February 12, 2021, https://www.netflix.com/title/80201728.

"Alpha Go," Wikipedia, accessed February 12, 2021, https://en.wikipedia.org/wiki/AlphaGo.

Chapter 9: Applied Change Management: From Stand-Alone Processes to Integrated Workflow

Heeringa, Jessica, Anne Mutti, Michael F Furukawa, Amanda Lechner, Kristin A Maurer, and Eugene Rich, "Horizontal and Vertical Integration of Health Care Providers: A Framework for Understanding Various Provider Organizational Structures," *International Journal of Integrative Care*, 2020, 20; 20(1): 2.

Chapter 10: Applied Change Management and Clinical Workflow

Koulopoulos, Tom, *The Workflow Imperative: Building Real World Business Solutions* (New York: Van Nostrand Reinhold, 1995).

"What Is Workflow?" Agency for Healthcare Research and Quality, accessed February 12, 2021, https://digital.ahrq.gov/health-it-tools-and-resources/evaluation-resources/workflow-assessment-health-it-toolkit/workflow.

"The Physicians Foundation 2020 Physician Survey: Part 1," The Physicians Foundation, August 18, 2020, https://physiciansfoundation.org/research-insights/2020physiciansurvey/.

Weed, Lawrence L., and Lincoln Weed, *Medicine in Denial* (CreateSpace Independent Publishing Platform, 2011).

Chapter 11: Applied Change Management and the Clinician

Shem, Samuel, *Man's 4th Best Hospital* (New York: Berkley, 2019).

Collier, Roger, "Electronic Health Records Contributing to Physician Burnout," *Canadian Medical Association Journal*, 2017, 189(45): E1405–E1406.

"Physician Supply," Wikipedia, accessed February 12, 2021, https://en.wikipedia.org/wiki/Physician_supply.

"An Interview with 'M,' a Pre-Med Student," conducted July 27, 2020.

Boudette, Neal E., "Inside Tesla's Audacious Push to Reinvent the Way Cars Are Made," *New York Times*, June 30, 2018, https://www.nytimes.com/2018/06/30/business/tesla-factory-musk.html.

Economy, Peter, "These 11 Elon Musk Quotes Will Inspire Your Success and Happiness," *Inc.*, accessed February 12, 2021, https://www.inc.com/peter-economy/11-elon-musk-quotes-that-will-push-you-to-achieve-impossible.html.

Chapter 12: Applied Change Management and the Patient

Aptowicz, Cristin O'Keefe, *Dr. Mutter's Marvels: A Tale of Intrigue and Innovation at the Dawn of Modern Medicine* (New York: Avery, 2014).

Shem, Samuel, *The House of God* (New York: G.P. Putnam, 1978).

Frellick, Marcia, "PCP Appointments Last 5 Minutes or Less in Half the World," Medscape, November 9, 2017, https://www.medscape.com/viewarticle/888270.

"Charles Holland Duell," Wikipedia, accessed February 12, 2021, https://en.wikipedia.org/wiki/Charles_Holland_Duell.

Mickle, Tripp, "How Tim Cook Made Apple His Own," *Wall Street Journal*, August 7, 2020, https://www.wsj.com/articles/tim-cook-apple-steve-jobs-trump-china-iphone-ipad-apps-smartphone-11596833902.

Chapter 13: You Say You Want a HIT Revolution

Economy, Peter, "These 11 Elon Musk Quotes Will Inspire Your Success and Happiness," *Inc.*, accessed February 12, 2021, https://

www.inc.com/peter-economy/11-elon-musk-quotes-that-will-push-you-to-achieve-impossible.html.

"Elon Musk," Wikipedia, accessed February 12, 2021, https://en.wikipedia.org/wiki/Elon_Musk.

Howard, Chris, "Reset Your Business Strategy in COVID-19 Recovery," Gartner, June 3, 2020, https://www.gartner.com/smarterwithgartner/reset-your-business-strategy-in-covid-19-recovery/.

Chapter 14: RHIT and Interoperability

Doyle, Arthur Conan, *The Valley of Fear* (New York: George H. Doran, 1915).

Johnson, Tiffany, "Brittany Kaiser, Author, Targeted," Wunderman Thompson, October 24, 2019, https://intelligence.wunderman-thompson.com/2019/10/brittany-kaiser-author-targeted.

"Recent Trends in Interoperability," https://www.healthit.gov/isa/united-states-core-data-interoperability-uscdi.

"How Doctors Feel About Electronic Health Records: National Physician Poll," The Harris Poll and Stanford Medicine, May 31, 2018, https://med.stanford.edu/content/dam/sm/ehr/documents/EHR-Poll-Presentation.pdf.

Chayefsky, Paddy, *The Hospital* (Film), 1971, https://www.imdb.com/title/tt0067217.

Chapter 15: RHIT and Quality

Bobrow, Emily, "Francis Collins Relies on Science and Faith," *Wall Street Journal*, August 7, 2020, https://www.wsj.com/articles/francis-collins-relies-on-science-and-faith-11596815855.

"Survey Uncovers Widespread Belief in 'Dangerous' Covid Conspiracy Theories," *Guardian*, accessed February 12, 2021, https://www.theguardian.com/world/2020/oct/26/survey-uncovers-widespread-belief-dangerous-covid-conspiracy-theories.

Institute of Medicine and Committee on Quality of Health Care in America, *Crossing the Quality Chasm* (Washington, DC: National Academies Press, 2001).

"Johann Wolfgang von Goethe Quotes," Goodreads Inc., accessed February 12, 2021, https://www.goodreads.com/quotes/9884-knowing-is-not-enough-we-must-apply-willing-is-not.

Nefiodow, Leo, "Kondratieff Cycles," accessed February 12, 2021, https://www.kondratieff.net/kondratieffcycles.

"What Is the Plan Do-Check-Act (PDCA) Cycle?" American Society for Quality, accessed February 12, 2021, https://asq.org/quality-resources/pdca-cycle.

Chapter 16: RHIT and Revolutionary Access

Liu, J.X., Y. Goryakin, A. Maeda, et al., "Global Health Workforce Labor Market Projections for 2030," Human Resources for Health, February 3, 2017, 15, 11.

Gawande, Atul, "We Can Solve the Coronavirus-Test Mess Now—If We Want To," *New Yorker*, September 2, 2020, https://www.newyorker.com/science/medical-dispatch/we-can-solve-the-coronavirus-test-mess-now-if-we-want-to.

Kurt, Daniel, and Khadija Khartit, "The Special Economic Impact of Pandemics," Investopedia, January 27, 2021, https://www.investopedia.com/special-economic-impact-of-pandemics-4800597.

Institute of Medicine, *The Role of Telehealth in an Evolving Health Care Environment: Workshop Summary* (Washington, DC: National Academies Press, 2012).

Chapter 17: RHIT and Outcomes

"I'm a doctor, not a…" Fandom, accessed February 12, 2021, https://memory-alpha.fandom.com/wiki/I%27m_a_doctor,_not_a…

"Seigfried Sassoon," Poetry Foundation, accessed February 12, 2021, https://www.poetryfoundation.org/poets/siegfried-sassoon.

"E. E. Cummings," Poetry Foundation, accessed February 12, 2021, https://www.poetryfoundation.org/poets/e-e-cummings.

Terlep, Sharon, "Clorox's New CEO Is Racing to Keep Wipes on Store Shelves," *Wall Street Journal*, September 25, 2020, https://www.wsj.com/articles/cloroxs-new-ceo-is-racing-to-keep-wipes-on-store-shelves-11601041820.

"Strategic Financial Planning," Healthcare Financial Management Association, 2018, https://www.cleverleyassociates.com/wp-content/uploads/2018/05/W2018_SFP_Welch.pdf.

International Consortium for Health Outcomes, https://www.ichom.org/. See also "Value-Based Healthcare: A Global Assessment," Economist Intelligence Unit, September 22, 2016, https://eiuperspectives.economist.com/healthcare/value-based-healthcare-global-assessment-1.

Lewis, Michael, *Moneyball* (New York: W. W. Norton, 2003).

Gay, Jason, "You Don't Have to Love the Tampa Bay Rays. You Just Shouldn't Hate Them," *Wall Street Journal*, October 22, 2020, https://www.wsj.com/articles/you-dont-have-to-love-the-tampa-bay-rays-you-just-shouldnt-hate-them-11603389232.

Chapter 19: The Connected, Adaptive Healthcare Organization

Forester, E. M. *Howards End* (London: Edward Arnold, 1910).

Acknowledgments

The famous songwriter Paul Simon starts his hit song, "Kodachrome," with these words:

> "When I think back on all the crap I learned in high
> school, it's a wonder I can think at all."

As much as I love the work of Mr. Simon, he got it a bit backwards for me. When I think back on all I learned in high school, especially out of the classroom, it is the primary reason I can think at all.

I entered South Shore High School as a sophomore in its first graduating class. The school opened offering only ninth and tenth grade classes. Over the next two years, South Shore High expanded to include the eleventh and twelfth grades. While most teenagers enter high school with some existing social structure—a sports team, club, student theater—my class was tasked with creating these high-school activities for ourselves. While others focused on recruiting a track team, setting up a student government, or forming a marching band, I helped create the student newspaper and was its first editor-in-chief. How did that happen? Let us just say my recruitment had something to do with a school boycott linked to desegragation and this line from an Elton John song: "And the *New York Times* said God was dead."

The faculty advisor to *Shorelines*, our student newspaper, was a kind, intelligent, strongly principled man named Ernie Seligmann. He was also my tenth-grade English teacher. Tall, thin, wearing a light grey/reddish beard and round glasses, he was curious, focused, and always interested in you. During my two years working on *Shorelines*, I learned so much about life from Ernie. This book is dedicated to him.

Joining me on my *Shorelines* journey were some amazing people who went on to achieve great success in their careers. Ernie made a lasting impression on them, too.

Beside every good doctor is an even better nurse. That applies to the hospital, the clinic, and the home. Beka Sfikas, the nurse beside me, also happens to be my wife. She cheered from the sidelines month after month as the book took form. Her support and homemade spanakopita made the toil during those many long nights easier.

Tom Koulopoulos, author and founder of the Delphi Group, encouraged me for years to write a book. Once I began, he was always there to advise me, all along the way. I am fortunate to have him as a colleague and friend.

When I thought about who might be willing to write the foreword for my book, John Halamka was at the top of my list. Few people have had such a lasting impact on healthcare information technology as has John, so when he agreed, I was thrilled. Thanks, John!

I am grateful to Mike Klein, founder of WTN Media and producer of the Digital Healthcare Conference, for his support, advice, and friendship. I am glad Mike has always encouraged me to reach high.

Several years ago, Boston University educator Joseph Restuccia invited me to deliver some guest lectures in his graduate-level course on healthcare information technology. Those guest lectures led to my teaching his course for two semesters while Joe tended to other academic responsibilities. It was a great experience and an important factor in writing this book. Thanks, Joe.

Paul Barach and I go back many years, due to our work in the field of quality and patient safety. When I reached out to Paul to interview him for my book, I never expected him to introduce me to half a dozen internationally–known giants in healthcare, whom I was able to interview. Thank you, Paul, for sharing your colleagues with me.

I want to thank the eighteen wise and knowledgeable experts in healthcare and information technology whose interviews appear throughout this book. They were gracious enough to give of their valuable time so I could explore their insights and share them with my readers.

Ian Chuang, a well-respected informaticist and friend, stepped in to help me identify a publisher, and I am grateful for his efforts.

My colleague and friend Derek Cyr provided wonderful insights into math and process control.

While most people dream of writing a book, no one writes one by themselves. For that reason, I want to thank my editor Jack B. Rochester. Over the many months Jack and I worked together, he has provided both guidance and support.

Christopher Cote did a fantastic job synthesizing complex ideas into meaningful images that led to the cover design and RHIT methodology graphic. Caitlin M. Park, who managed the entire editorial interview process, clearly ranks among the most talented and versatile of editors. Michael Fedison wore two hats, acting as both copyeditor and proofreader, and got the job done with amazing attention to detail. Victoria "Tori" Merkle is the consummate master of so many publishing talents, including publicity and marketing.

Eddie Vincent was kind enough to share his vast experience in book publishing to help me get my book into reader's hand. I am grateful to the professionals at Books International—Eric Moar,

Carmen Jackson, Mike Whalen, and Bill Clockel—for their excellence in post-production, printing, and distribution.

Fortunately, I had talented audio arts professionals, James Delhauer, Hannah Edelson, and Christopher Moore, voiceover actors all, and Ruby Fink pulling their recordings together to produce my audiobook.

I want to thank Grace Chu for her smiling hospitality and kindness —and for serving my favorite Earl Grey tea.

I am also very grateful to Jose Sosa, Paul Reagan, Cliff Matthews, and Ray Goepfrich for being such good friends.

I want to honor the writers, editors, and publishers of the *New York Times,* who over the years have provided me with a broad education in science, history, culture, and politics, which far exceeded anything I could have ever learned in a classroom.

I also wish to acknowledge the world's journalists who have sacrificed so much to bring us facts and truth, demonstrating daily the value of a free press. The world is a more just, safe, and livable place because of them.

–30–

Barry P. Chaiken
Boston, MA
May 6, 2021

About the Author

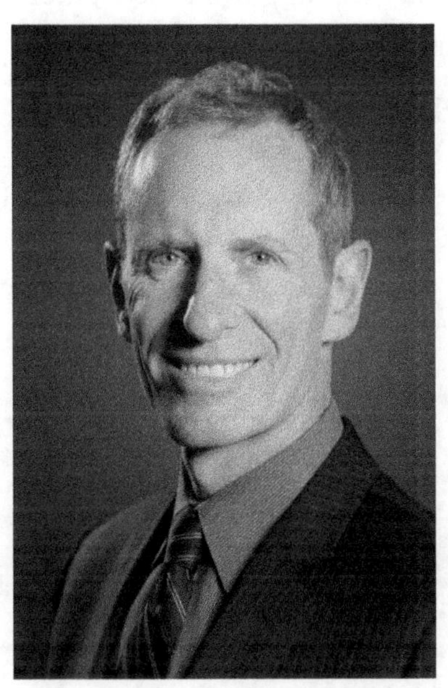

Barry P. Chaiken, MD, MPH has over 25 years' experience in healthcare information technology, clinical transformation, and business intelligence. He provides thought leadership and strategic and analytics assessments in healthcare information technology, quality of care, clinical change management, and business development. Chaiken has worked with, the NIH, Tableau/Salesforce, Infor, McKesson, UK National Health Service, Boston University, and others.

Chaiken served as a healthcare advisory board member to numerous organizations as head of DocsNetwork, his own boutique healthcare IT consulting company. He has served as guest lecturer and consultant on topics including patient safety, clinician adoption of information technology, quality improvement, and healthcare analytics. Chaiken assisted hospitals and technology firms in the creation of medical software products and services. He has delivered more than 60 CME lectures and was Conference Chair of the annual Digital Healthcare Conference.

Chaiken served as a Board member (2006-2010), Board Liaison to HIMSS Europe (2006-2009), and Board Chair (2009-2010), and continues his involvement as a Fellow of HIMSS. He is an Overseas Fellow of the Royal Society of Medicine.

Chaiken is board certified in General Preventive Medicine and Public Health. He received his medical degree from Downstate Medical Center and his MPH degree from the Harvard School of Public Health. He acquired his specialty training from the Centers for Disease Control as an Epidemic Intelligence Service officer and from the NJ Department of Health as a preventive medicine resident.